# AN *atlas* OF *dental* CARIES

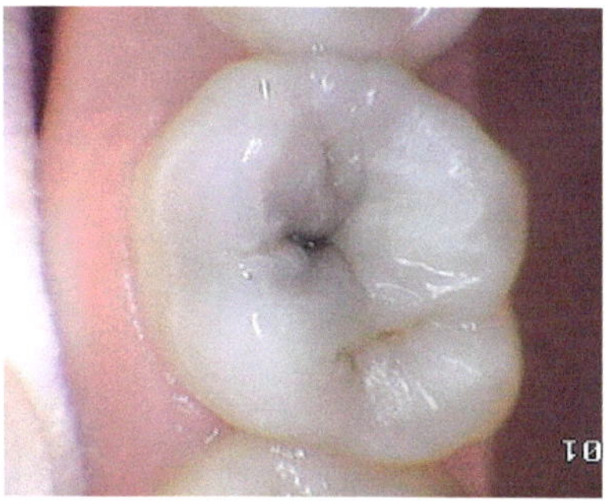

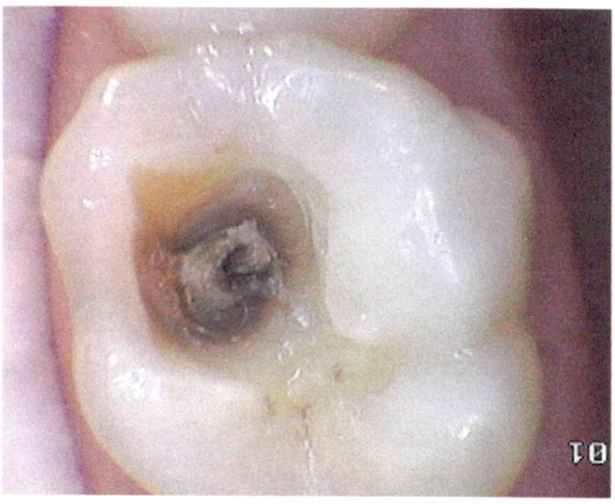

## A Pictorial For Dental Students and Dentists

Dr. Nazir A Mahomed

An Atlas of Dental Caries: A Pictorial For Dental Students and Dentists


ISBN: 978-1-922354-38-9 (paperback)

Dental Education Series Book One

For educational resources for dental students and junior dentists, visit www.mydentaleducation.com



Published in Australia by Dr. Nazir A Mahomed and InHouse Publishing.
www.inhousepublishing.com.au

Printed in Australia by InHouse Print & Design.

INHOUSE PTY LTD PUBLISHING

I would like to thank my nephew, Zubair Khatry, for his expertise and the time he spent in guiding me with this book, and Chrisstie and Caroline at InHouse Publishing for bringing the work to completion.

I give special thanks to my lovely wife, Hawa, and children, Razia and Ziyaad, for their patience, support and encouragement over the years as I put the manuscript together. I love you all so much.

I thank Almighty God for all he has blessed me with and for the opportunity to pass on my knowledge to future generations.

I dedicate this book to all students of dentistry. These are exciting times as our profession gallops ahead with advances in technology and materials. Enjoy the ride!

## DISCLAIMER

The author has practised as a general dental practitioner for close on 40 years. The contents of this book are based on his personal professional experiences and any advice given is general in nature. He does not profess to be an expert in the field of caries. This Atlas of Dental Caries is a general guide and any suggested treatments or preventive measures are not intended to be a substitute for the reader's own training on diagnosis and treatment planning. Any treatment decisions should be based on the reader's own professional judgement. Any errors or omissions are unintentional. Neither the author nor the publisher can be held responsible any loss, injury or claim arising from the use or misuse of the information contained in this book.

# *dental* INDEX

# Introduction

Dental caries is one of the most common diseases of the human body. A high percentage of a general dentist's time is taken up in attending to this dental caries once it has penetrated the outer enamel layer, and in the repair work that is required in the ensuing years due to restorations breaking or further breakdown of tooth structure occurring in heavily restored teeth.

Teeth are the hardest structure in the body and will withstand a lot of insult. For them to develop caries the patient must be doing quite a lot of things wrong. There are three main areas where teeth get caries, one being in the pitted and fissured biting surfaces of the molars, the other being in areas where the teeth touch each other, and the third being at or near the gum lines of the lip/cheek-side, and tongue/palate-side of the teeth.

The International Caries Classification and Management System (ICCMS) is a standard that is taught to dental students as a guide for the management of teeth affected by dental caries. As a student and dentist, you have to recognize that no two patients are the same, and that dental caries is a multifactorial process. The tooth simply does not collapse in a heap overnight. You may see a lesion on a tooth where at some stage decalcification occurred, caries started, then conditions changed and the tooth re-hardened. You need to consider the condition of the mouth and all the aetiological factors to assist you in deciding whether you will leave this lesion alone and monitor it over time, or step in, cut away tooth structure and fill the cavity.

You will come across situations of an adult patient who it seems never cleans, does not know what a tooth brush is, and their gums are healthy and there are no cavities, and yet another patient cleans so well but there is always a low grade chronic gum problem with bleeding and with cavities developing every so often.

At other times you will see that within the same family there will be the diligent child who eats all the right food, does not snack between meals, cleans his/her teeth well, does absolutely everything by the book, and develops cavities, and then on the other hand you have a similar age sibling, eats all the wrong food, the mouth barely sees a toothbrush, and never gets cavities.

As you go through this atlas, think "prevention" and "minimal intervention". It is imperative that you only cut away tooth structure as a last resort. Of course with a tooth with large areas of dental caries you have no choice. But it is for those borderline cases that you must take a step back and decide carefully whether you will cut into the tooth or whether you will do your level best to stabilize that lesion and perhaps even reverse the decalcification using some of the myriad of preventive tools we have at our disposal. Look at the patient holistically, his/her age, oral hygiene, diet, saliva and motivation.

Most of all remember that the moment you pick up your handpiece to drill, you start a cycle that in some patients can lead to repeated breakdown and repeated fillings on the same tooth, getting bigger progressively, eventually needing a crown, maybe even endodontic treatment and finally tooth loss. Could it all have been avoided? Could you have done things differently? In hindsight, was your approach the best one? You have a lot in your arsenal to help teeth: fluoride, improved oral hygiene through oral hygiene instruction, use of plaque disclosing tablets, use of topical fluoride and lower concentrations of the same in daily or weekly rinses, antibacterial mouth rinses, dietary investigation and advice, resin infiltration, fissure sealants, and CPP-ACP creams, to mention just a few.

Your patient is putting their absolute trust in you, hence be proactive in helping them. Talk to your patients in simple language they can understand, and demonstrate to them how to brush and floss effectively. It is in your power to break them out of a cycle of repeated breakdown of their teeth, of new cavities forming with regularity and so save their teeth from the downhill slope that they are on.

Over the years I have seen dental students in all years of study, from those seeing patients for the first time through to final year students who are about to graduate, struggle in deciding what to fill and what not to, when to step in and when not to. Sometimes it may simply be stained fissures on molars, or it may be staining around an old composite resin filling, or craze lines on upper incisors, or some "ditching" around a large 65 year old occlusal amalgam filling on an 80 year old patient..... more than likely in each of these situations you would do nothing.

This struggle that I see students of dentistry have with detecting dental caries and in deciding how to proceed is what has prompted me to write this book, An Atlas Of Dental Caries, that derives from lectures I have delivered to dental students. There are over 200 high resolution photographs of teeth and bitewing radiographs. In looking at picture after picture and X-ray after X-ray, I would hope that the contents of this atlas will assist all of you to detect caries more easily and help you to discern when to step in and know what to do, and also when to leave things alone and rather monitor the patient over time. For tooth notations, the International Dental Federation (FDI) tooth numbering system has been used throughout this book.

Students of dentistry today are at the cusp of great things. There are rapid technological advances in materials and techniques. Patients are living longer; they are keeping their teeth for longer and are more dentally aware. At the same time there are increasing numbers of the very old and infirm, many now who cannot look after themselves as well as in the past or care for their teeth like they used to. Some of these patients, sadly, will present with rapid breakdown, or with many areas of cemental caries. This atlas addresses these issues and will, I hope, be a reference guide to assist you in recognising diseased tooth structure and guide you in your decision making.

Dr. Nazir Mahomed
BDS (Birmingham, 1980)

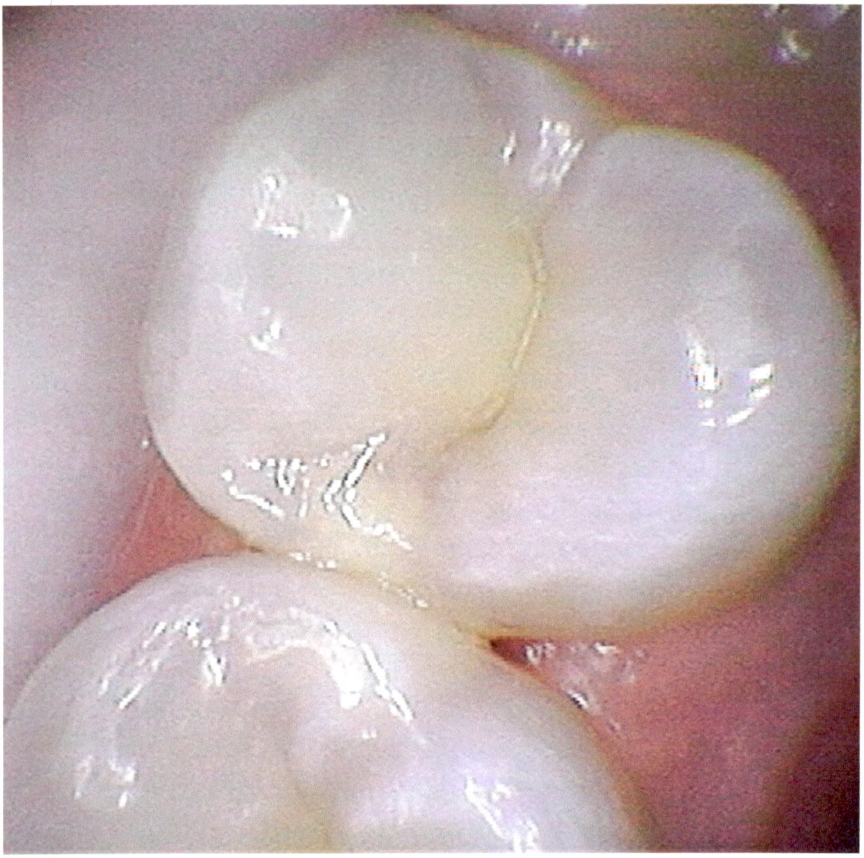

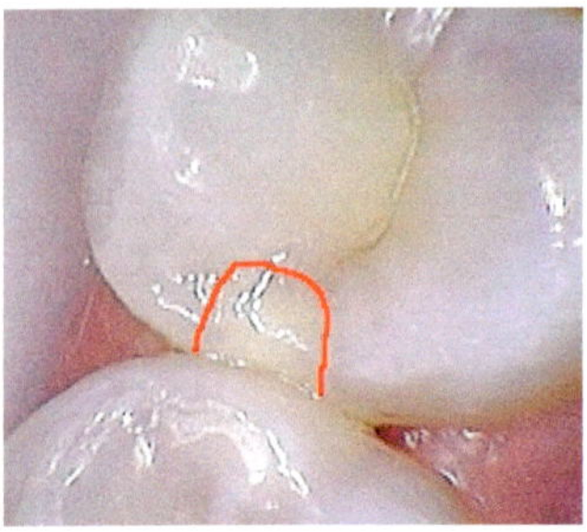

See the yellow discolouration in 14D? This is caries that has penetrated the enamel layer and is spreading into dentine. You must dry the teeth to detect those subtle colour changes that indicate dental caries.

# Occlusal CARIES

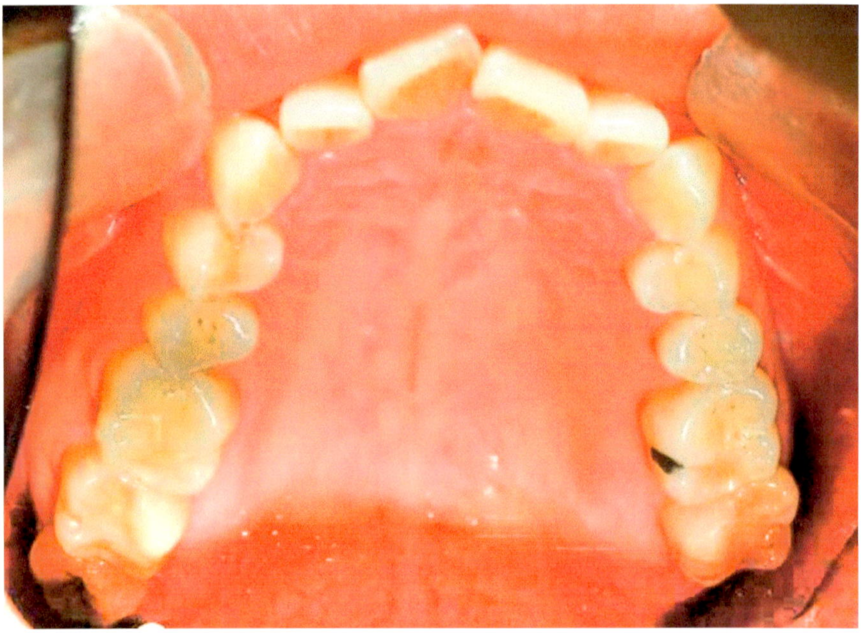

Consider age, oral hygiene and the periodontal/gingival health. This patient has good oral hygiene and the gingival health is good. The teeth look fine and no problems are evident. If you are seeing this patient for the first time you might want to take bitewing radiographs if you suspect interproximal caries.

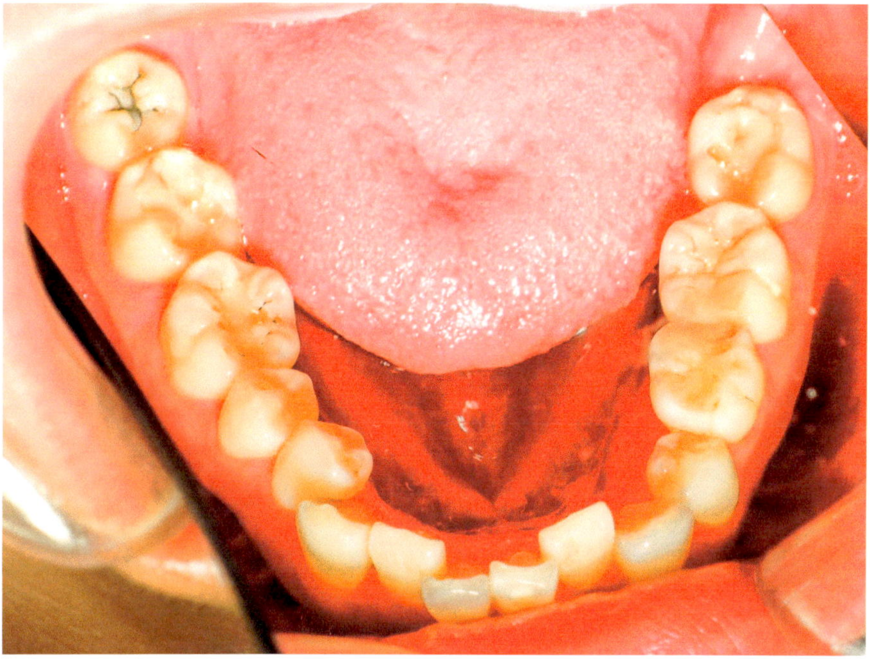

The 75DO restoration needs assessment clinically and radiographically. Quite likely the 35 is congenitally absent and, unless the 75 is going to be removed for orthodontic or implant reasons, you want to ensure the tooth is restored and retained long term.

48 with moderately deep occlusal caries, many years old. The surface is still intact and the fissures may not be sticky in this case, but it is the changes in the colour of the tooth around the fissures that should alert you to suspect the tooth is carious.

This page and the next two pages.

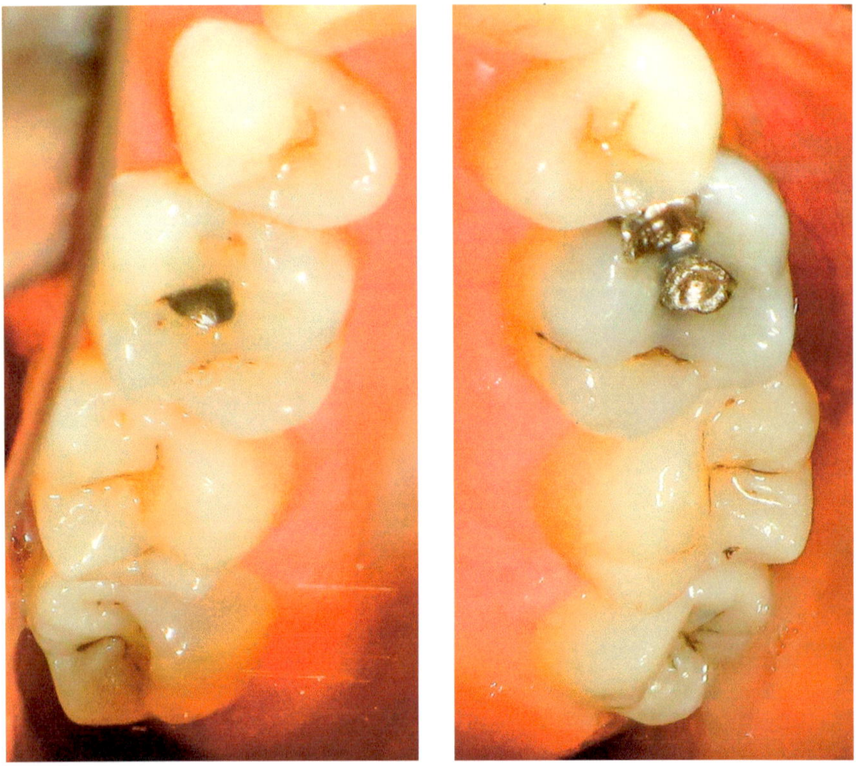

Old amalgam fillings. No caries.

The grey shadowing around the amalgam filling in 26 is due to diffusion of material into tooth structure, and often because the filling is larger internally than it is on the surface (see the left bitewing radiograph page 6)

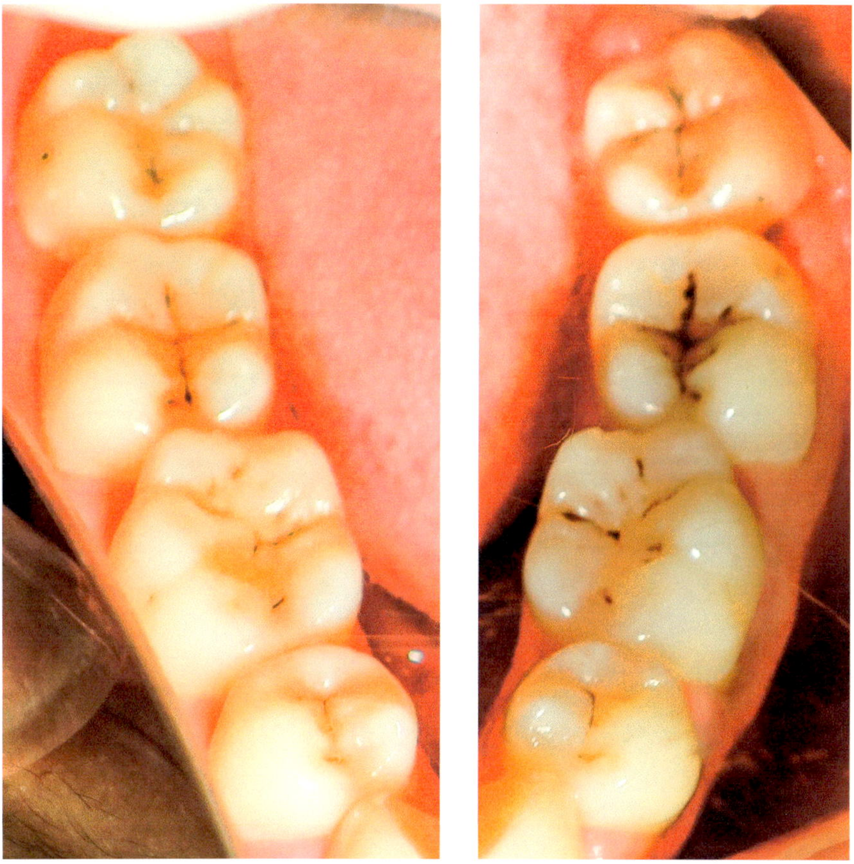

Stained pits and fissures, no caries.

There is no discolouration peripheral to these shallow pits and fissures. Check for stickiness of the fissures in 37 and 38 with an explorer. See bitewing radiographs next page.

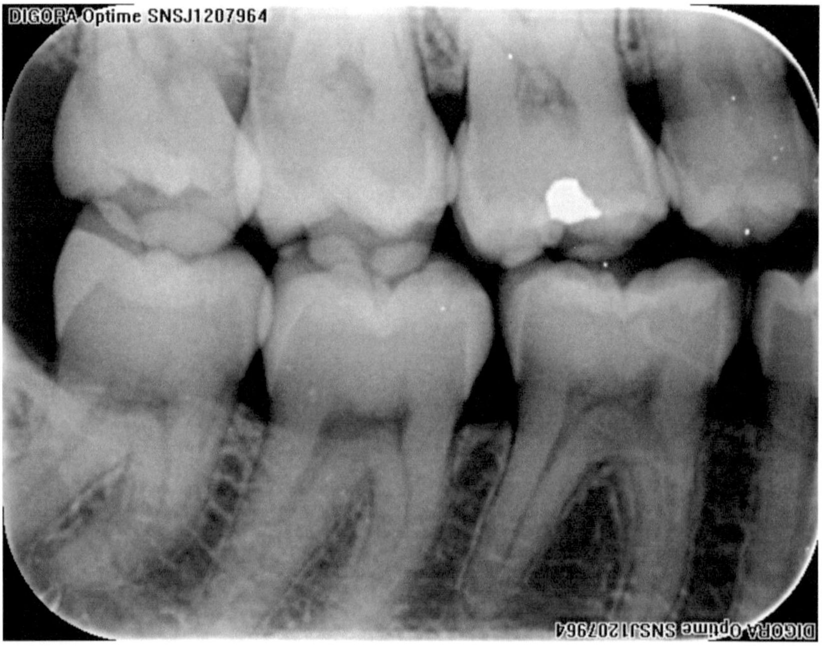


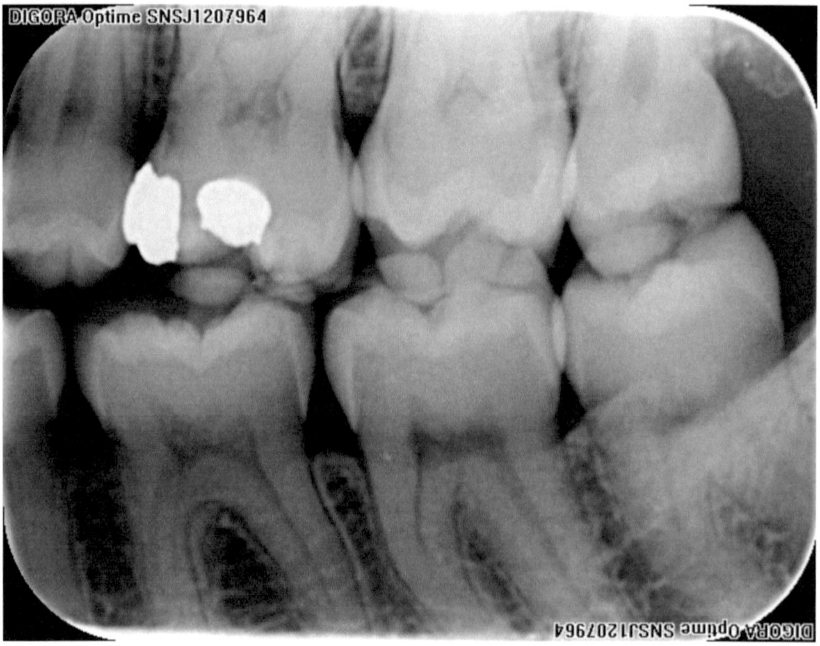


Right and left bitewing radiographs of the pages just seen – no caries. These amalgam fillings have been there for 37 years.

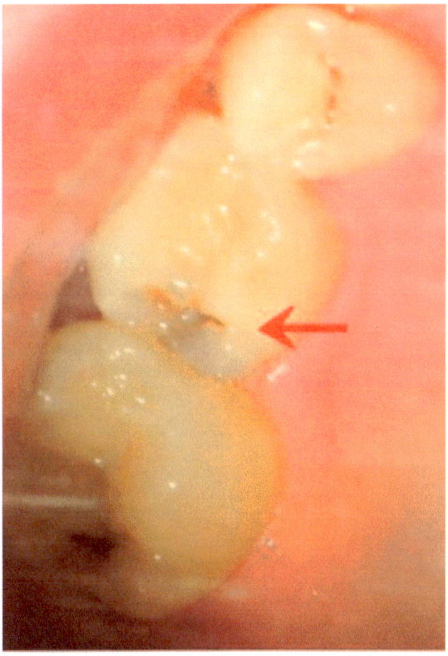

55D and 16O caries with spread into dentine.

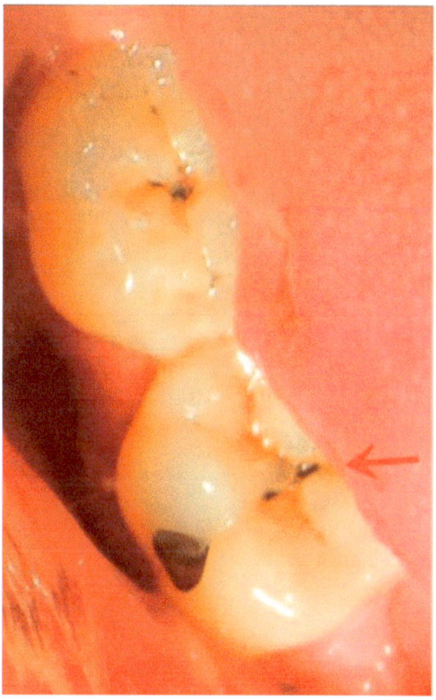

46O has occlusal caries through a deep area in the fissures, seen by colour changes and by probing.

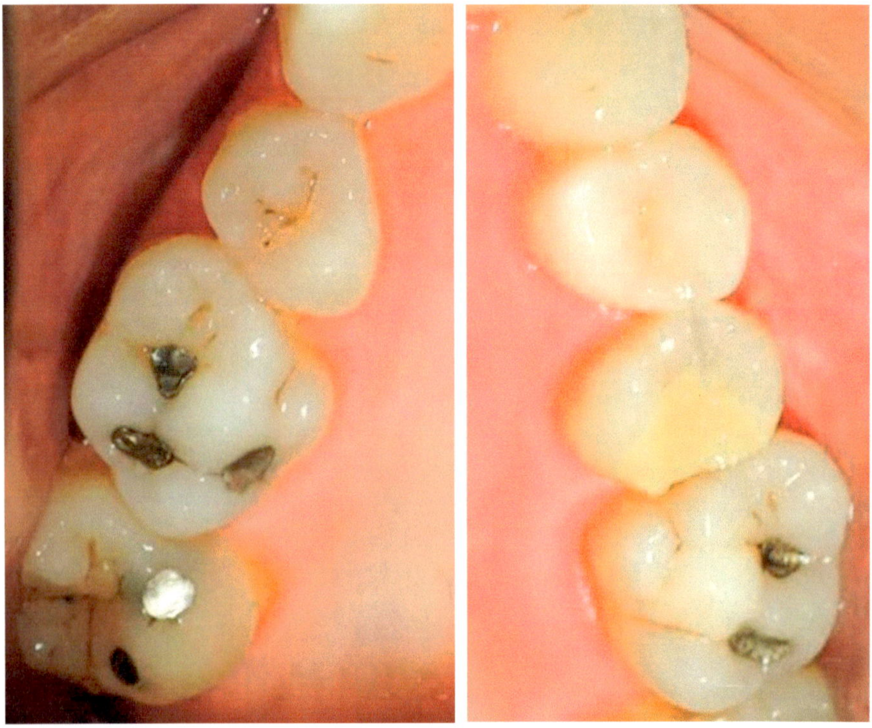

Good oral hygiene. Gingival health is good. Old fillings, all look fine. Everything is stable. 25 appears to have a GIC dressing with breakdown in the distal aspect, needs replacing with a more permanent restoration.

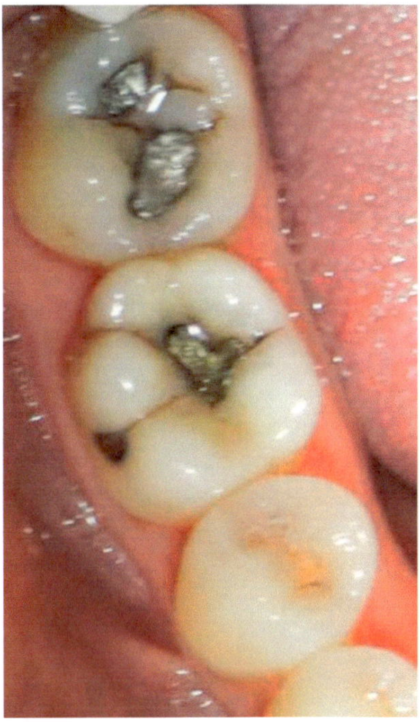

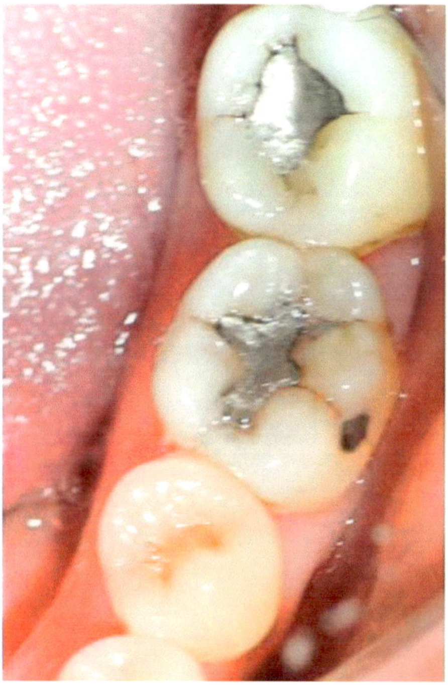

Visually and clinically no caries is suspected. It would be prudent to take two bitewing radiographs to look at how things are beneath these amalgam fillings.

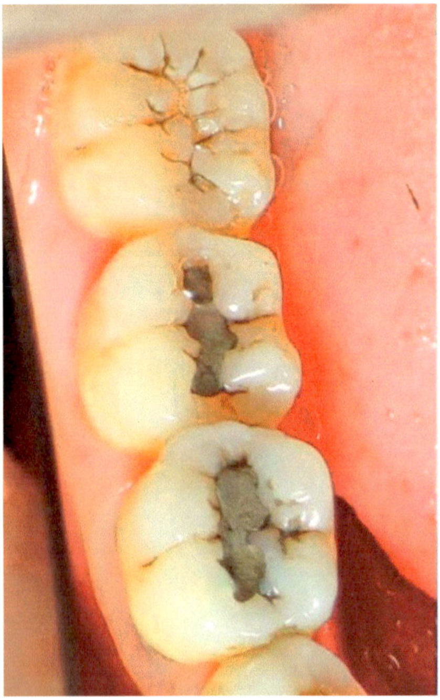

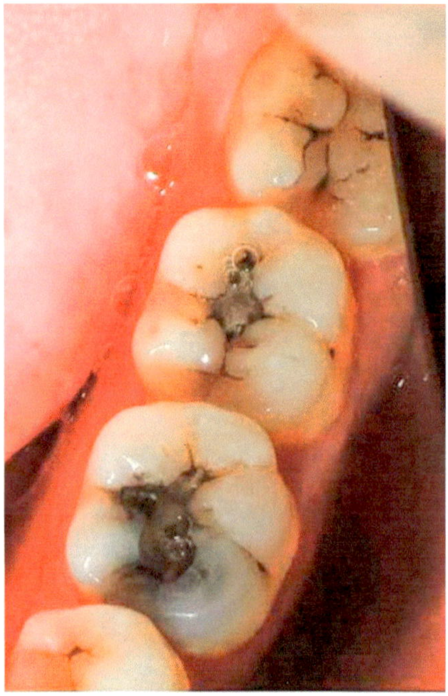

37, 38, 46, 47 and 48 are fine.

On 36 the amalgam filling appears to be very wide internally in the mesio-occluso-buccal area, resulting in grey staining showing through thin enamel. It would be prudent to take a left bitewing radiograph to check on 36.

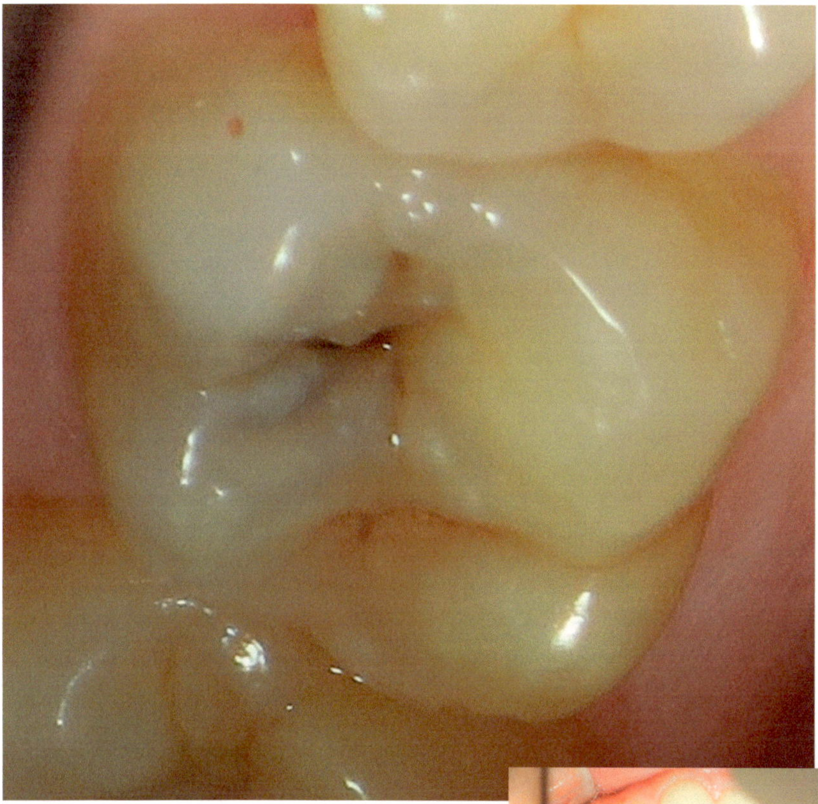

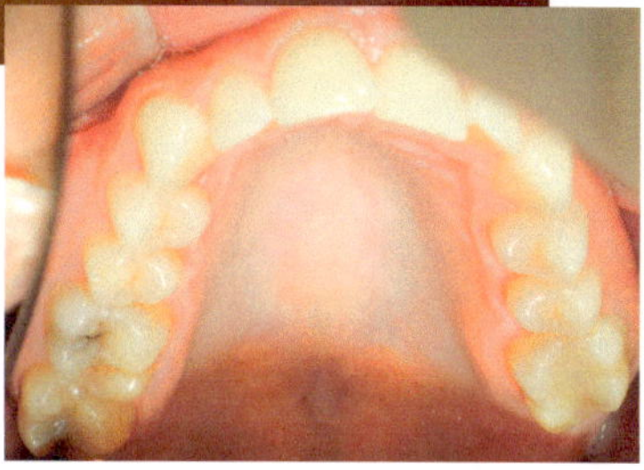

16 has occlural caries. See all the colour changes internally around the mesial fissure, compared to the healthy distal fissure?

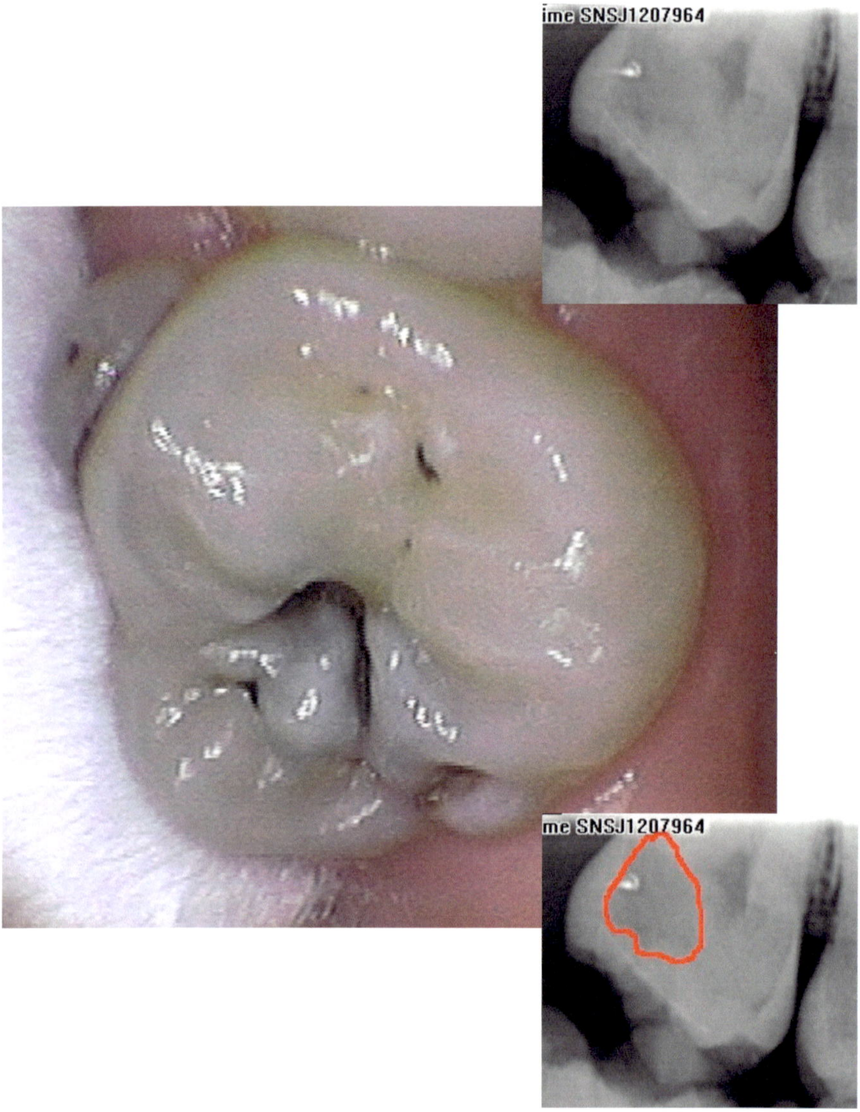


Very deep occlusal caries in 17. Note the colour changes in the tooth in the distal half, and the extent of the caries, outlined on the x-ray. Judging by the dark colour in the fissures, this has been caries spreading gradually over many years.

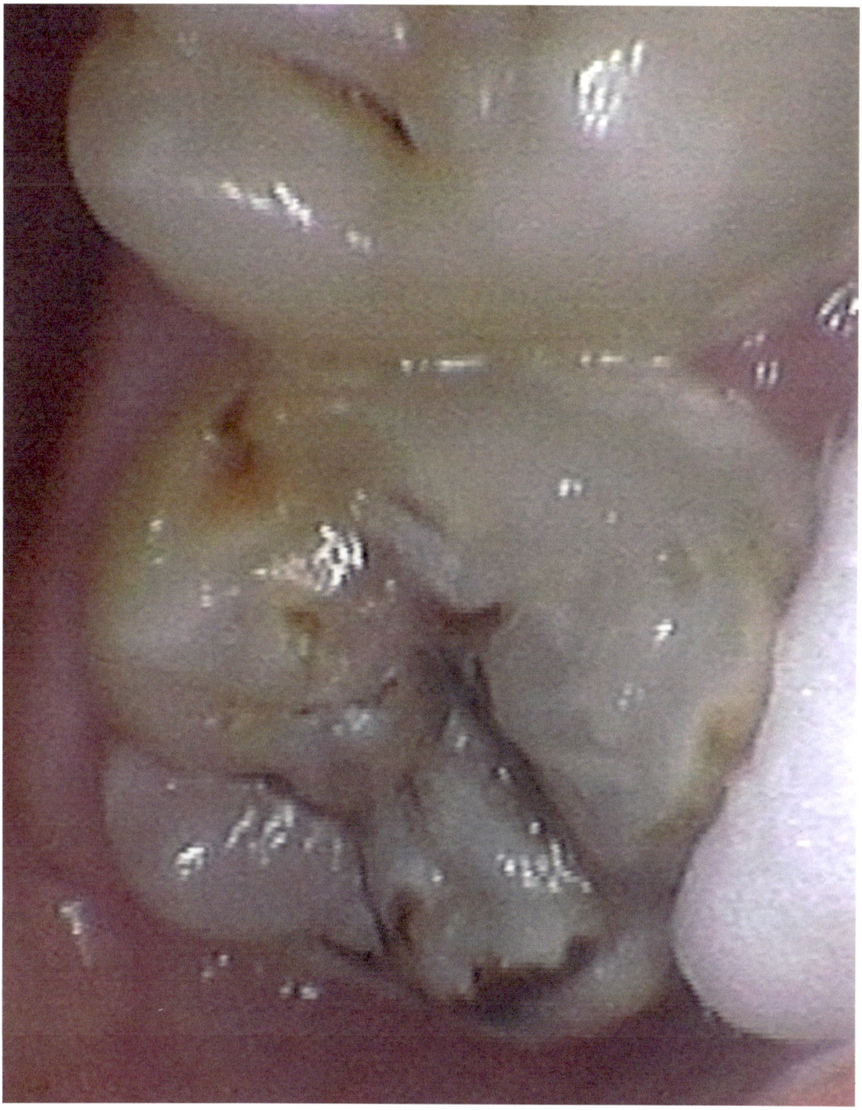

Looking at the distal tilt of this 27, it has been hard for the patient to clean. There are deep fissures and extensive discolouration. Beneath the occlusal enamel you will find a lot of caries. See also pages 14 and 15.

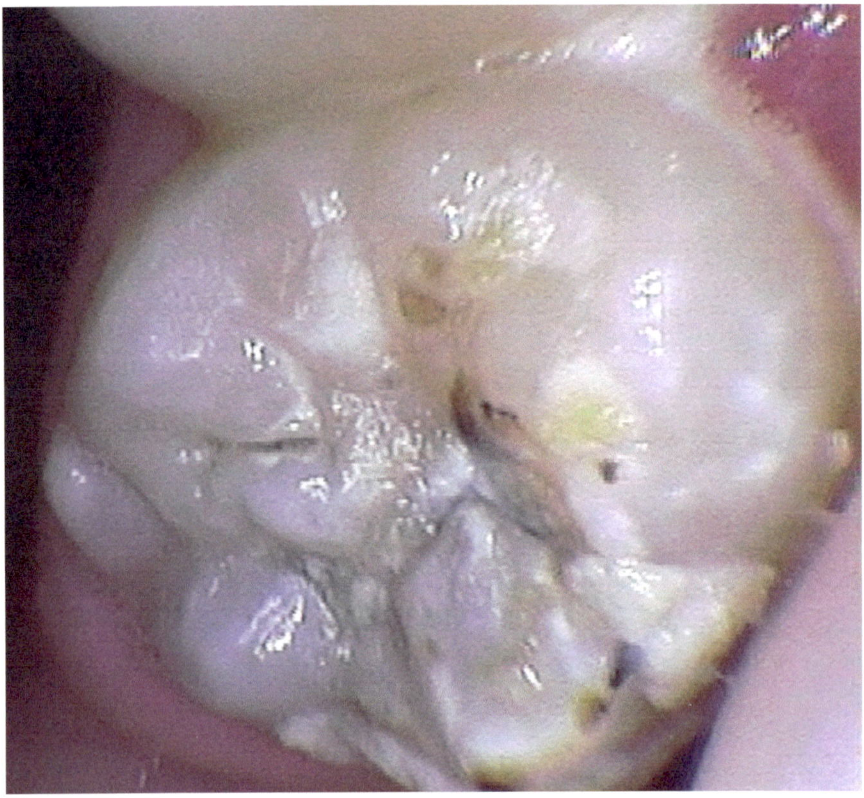

The surface has remained intact but you can expect to find extensive caries beneath it.

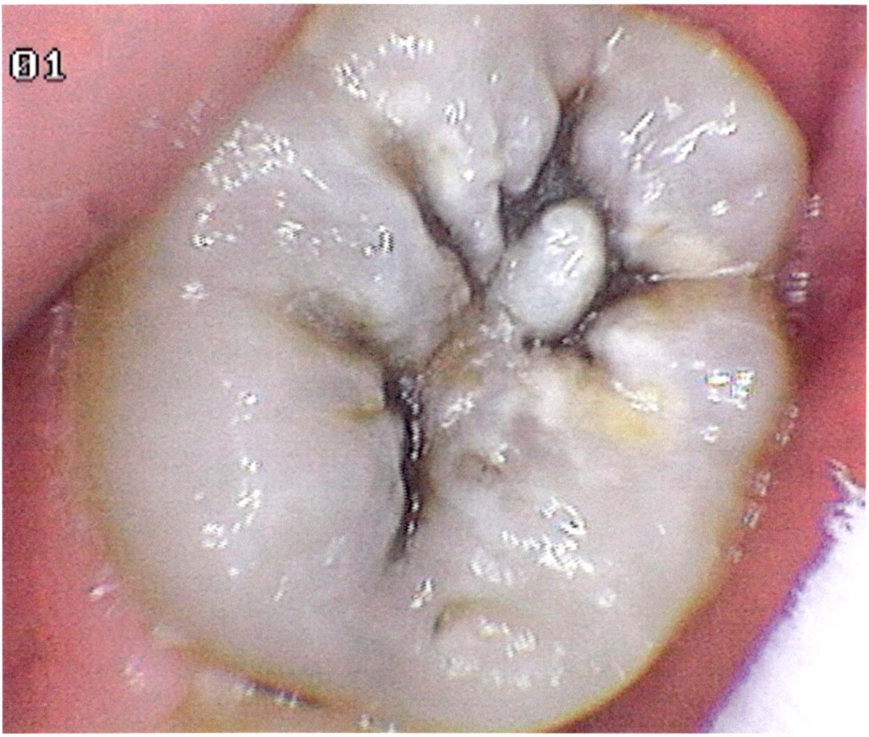


The surface has remained intact but you can expect to find extensive caries beneath it.

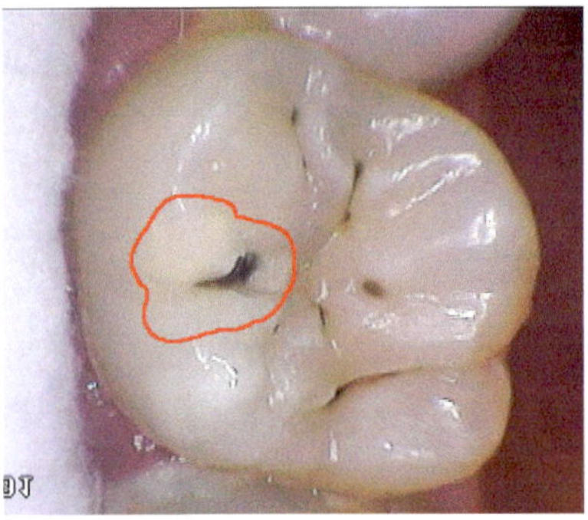

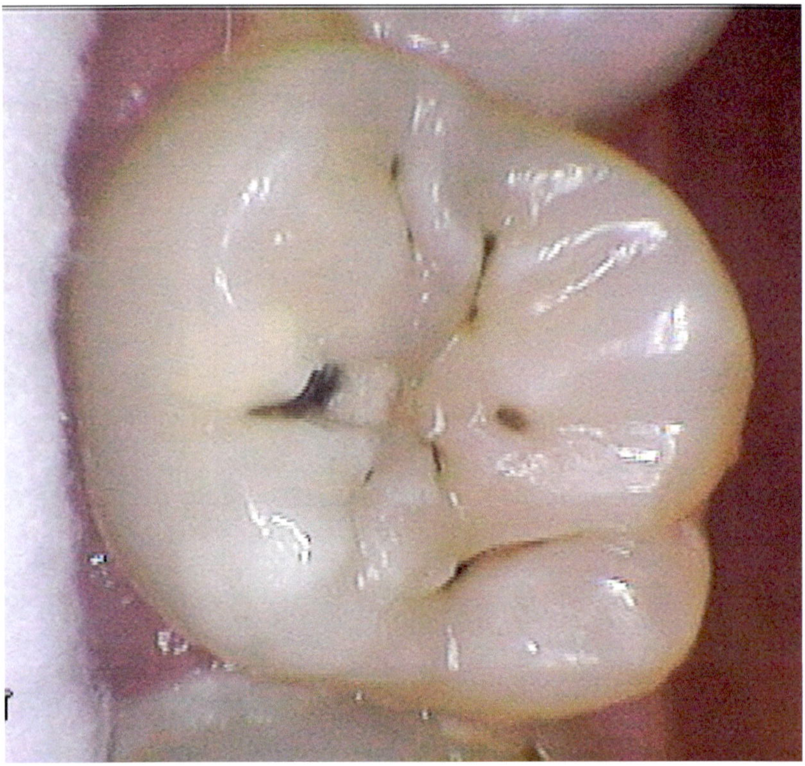

Has deep caries in the area outlined – see the colour changes in the enamel and the fissure broken open?

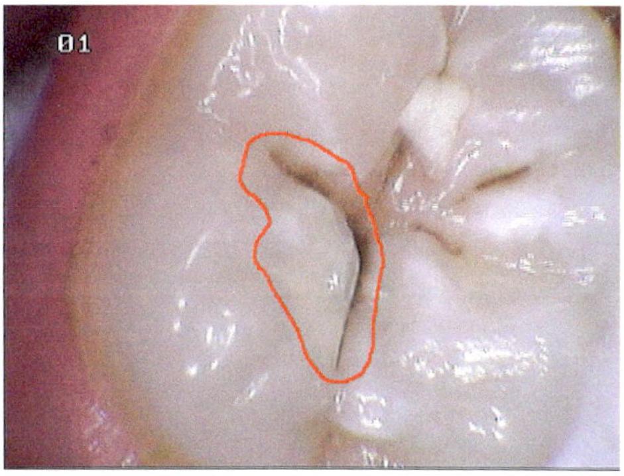


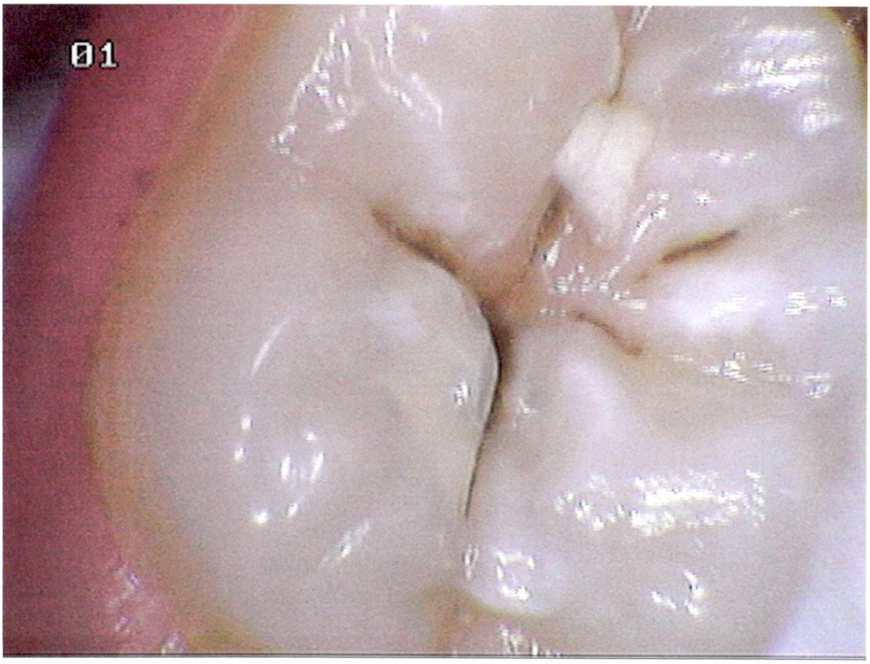


The main area of caries is outlined – see the creamy to yellow colour changes in the tooth? Also seen is a remnant of a fissure sealant on the distal part of the fissure.

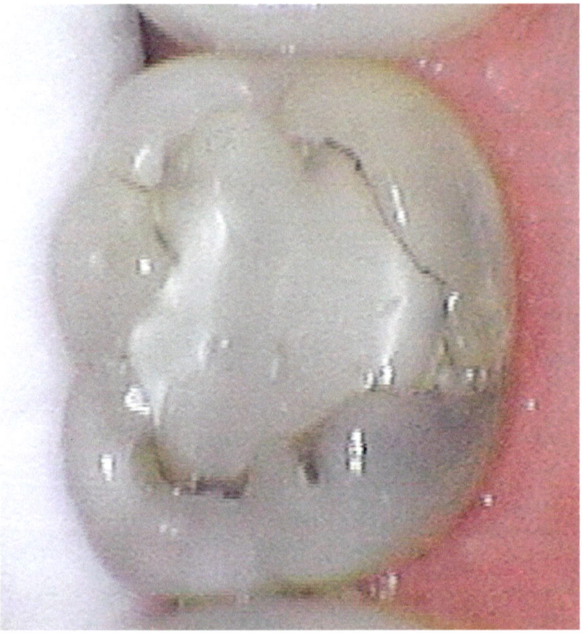

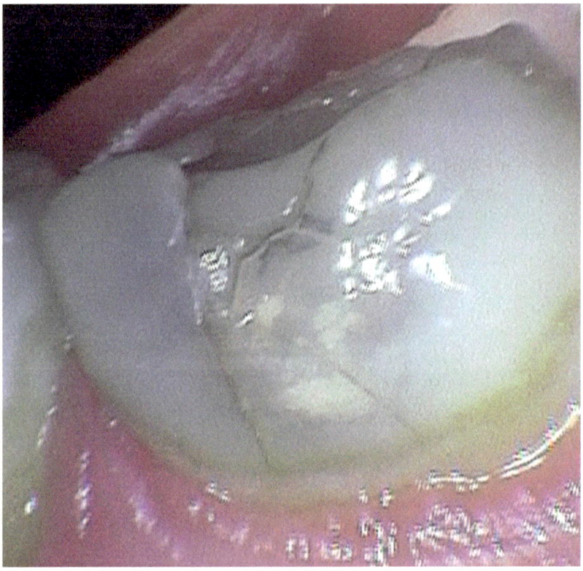

Deep caries in 36 beneath and buccal to a composite resin filling.

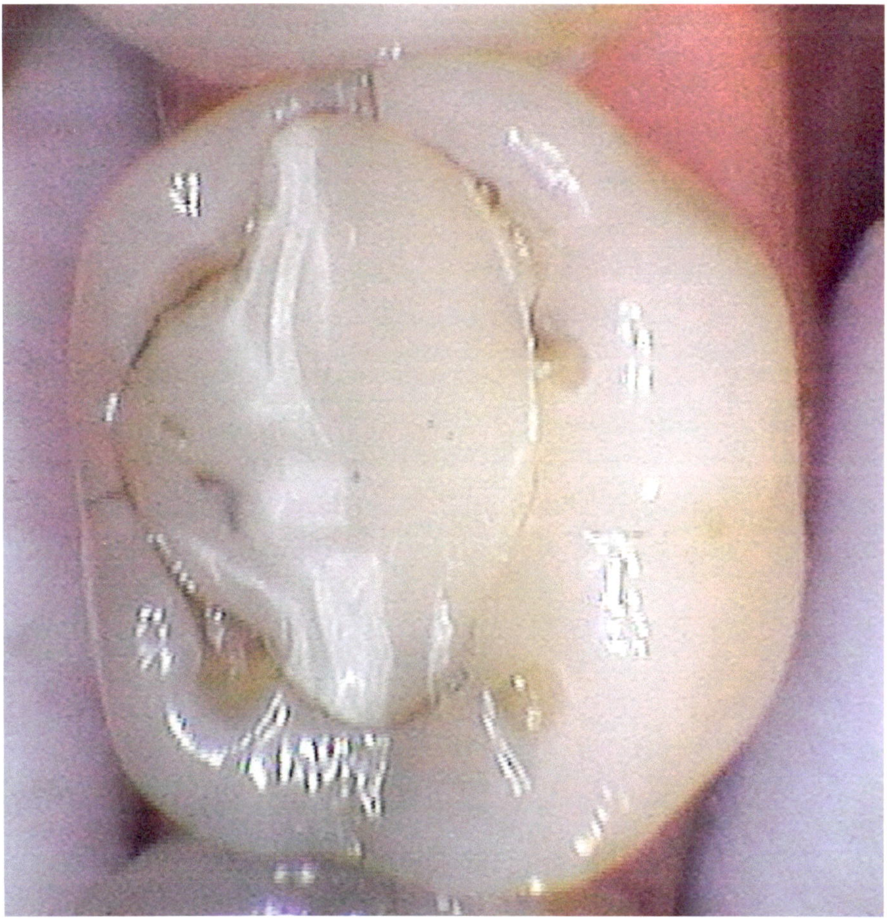

No caries. Wear facets an indication of strong chewing forces or parafunction, and possibly some erosion at play.

This page and the next three pages.

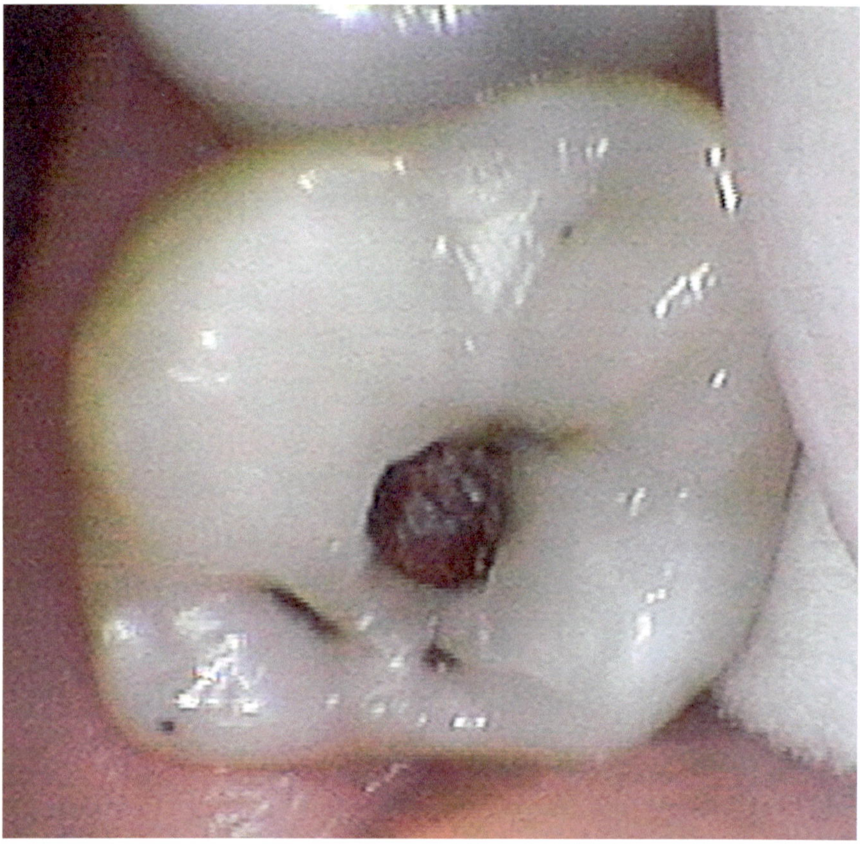

Deep occlusal caries in 27 (bitewing x-ray next page).

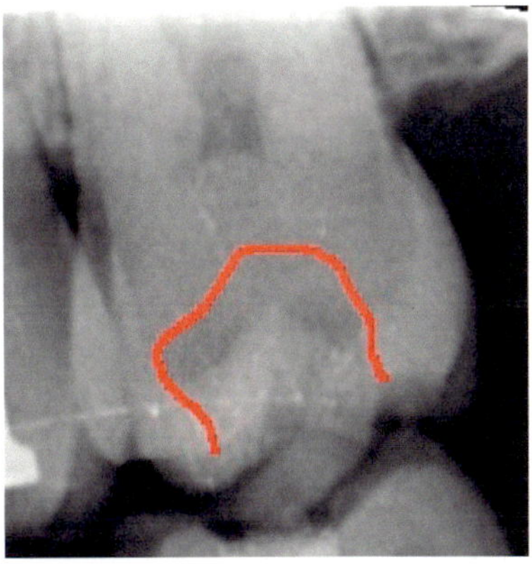

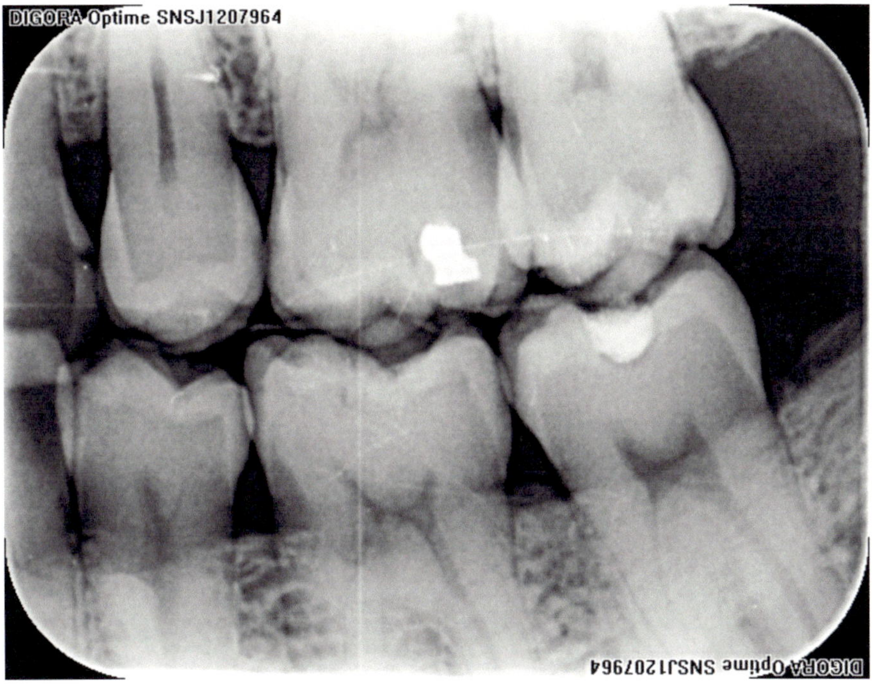


Moderately deep occlusal caries in 27, with the probable extent of the caries outlined.

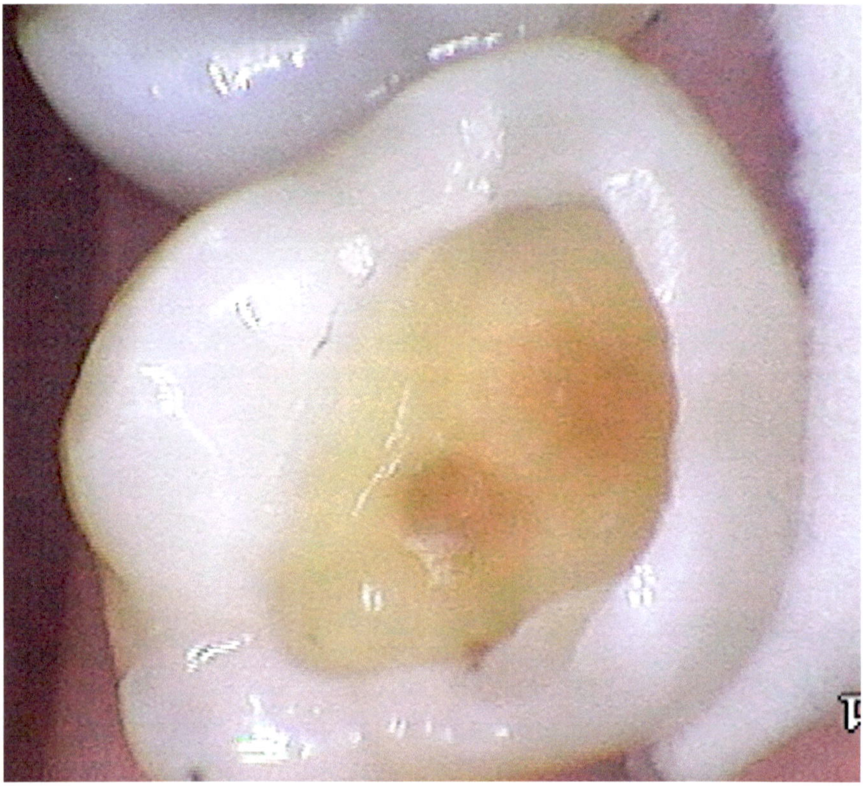

The cavity is caries-free.

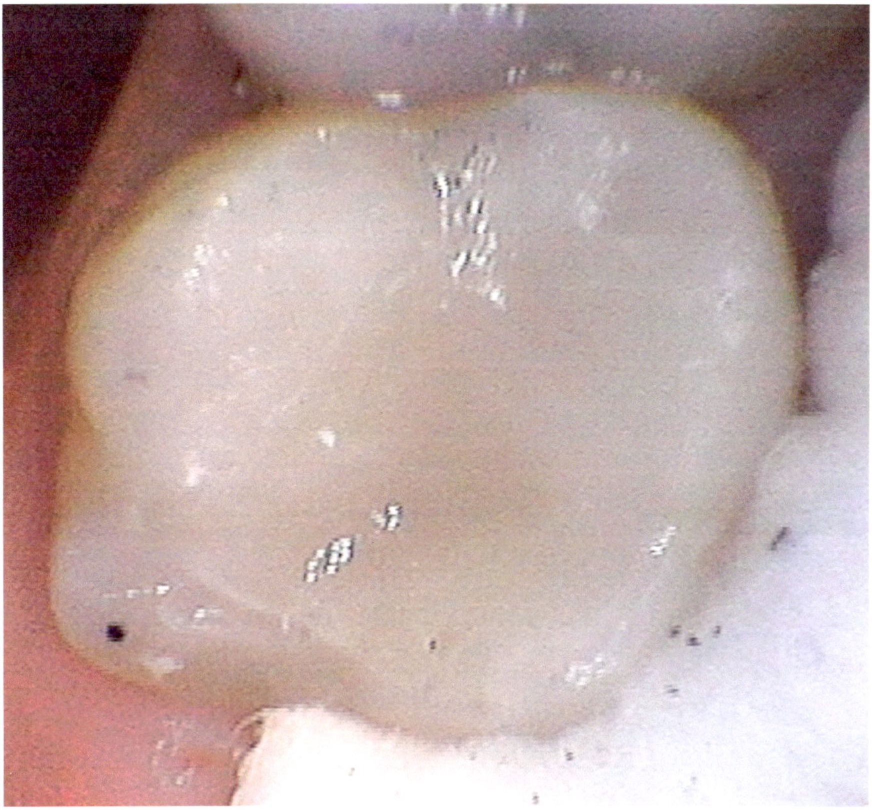

The cavity restored.

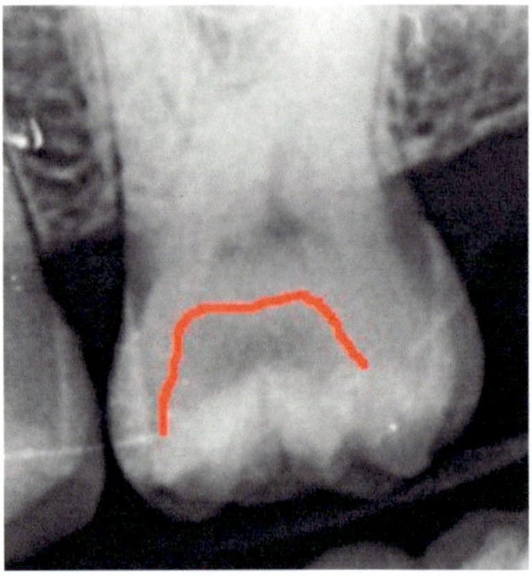

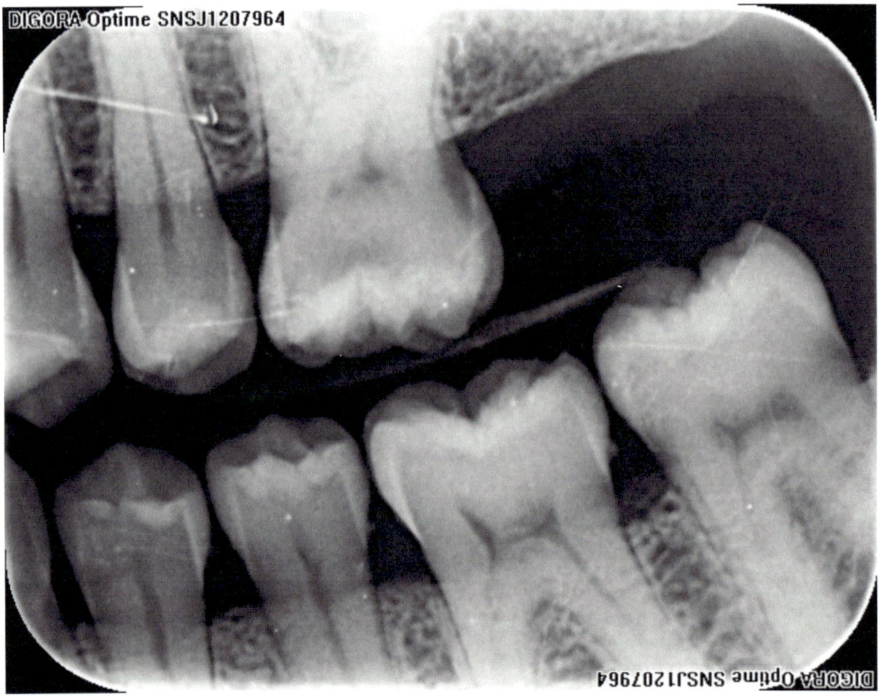


Very deep occlusal caries in 26. The extent of the caries is usually 30% larger than what the radiograph shows.

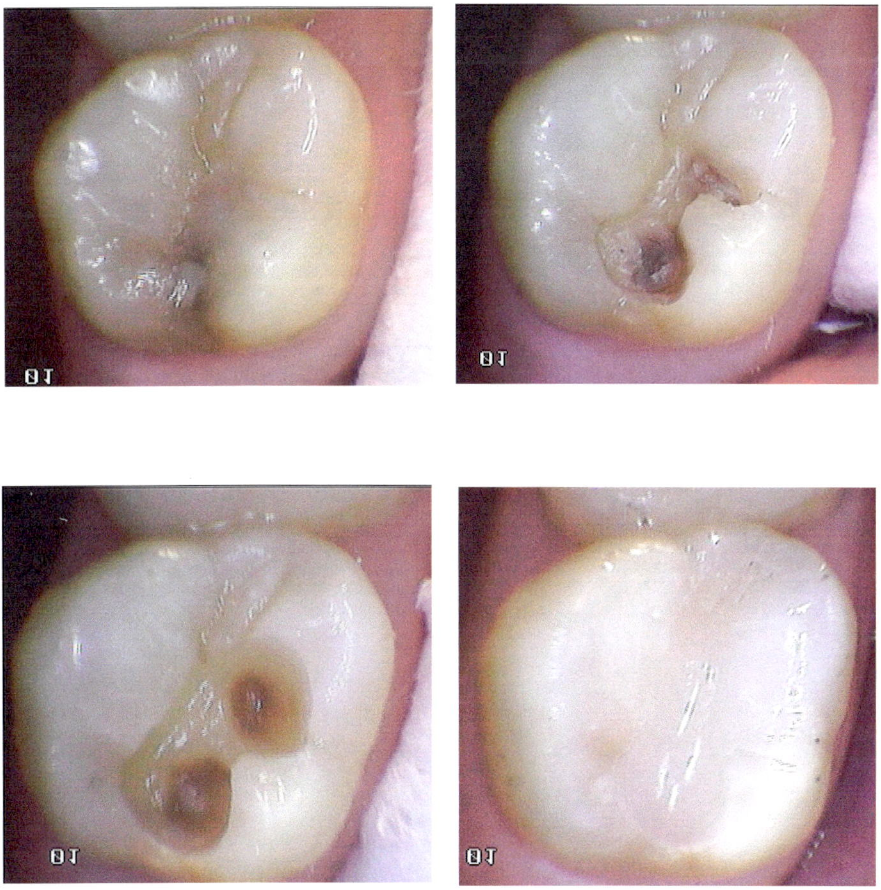

27 with occlusal caries that had been covered over by a fissure sealant. Extensive discolouration seen beneath the enamel surface.

This page and the next four pages.

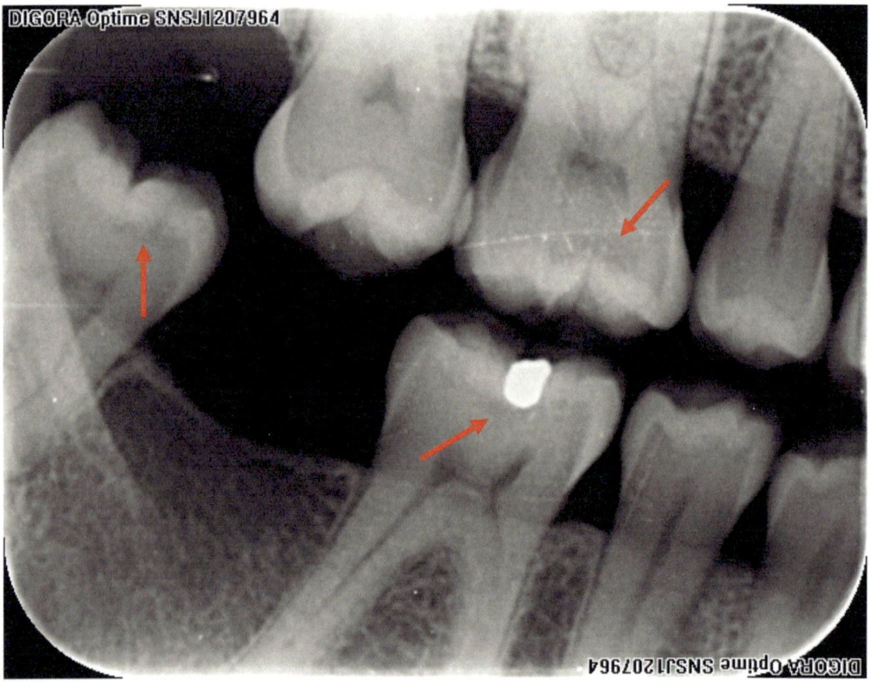


Deep occlusal caries in 16. Occlusal caries in 46 and 48.

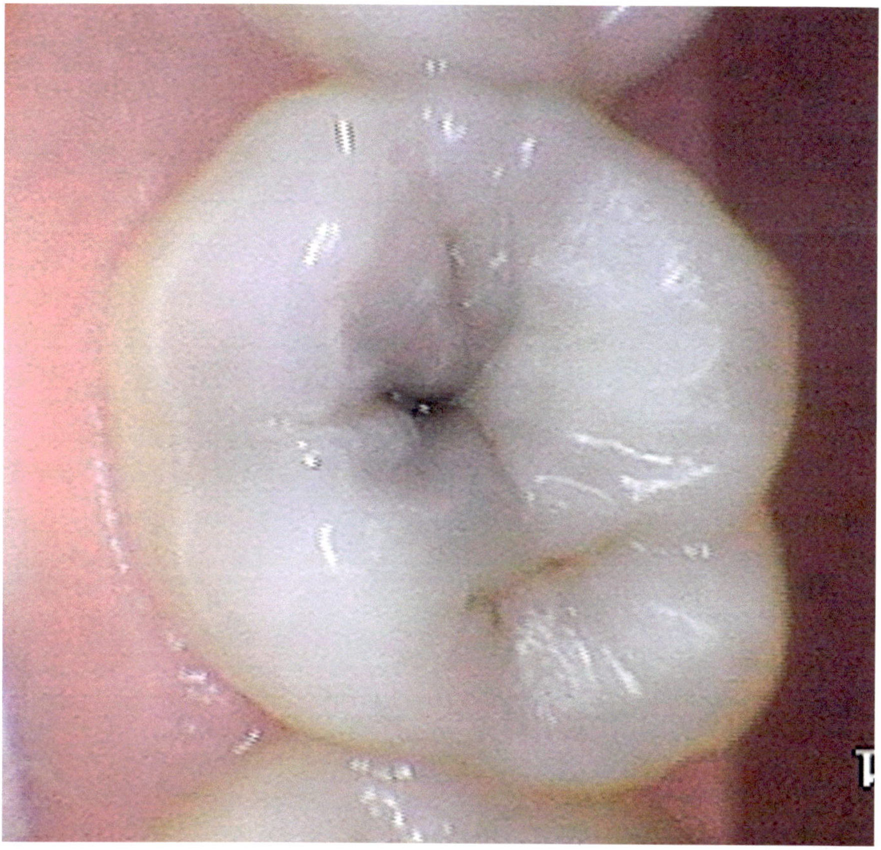

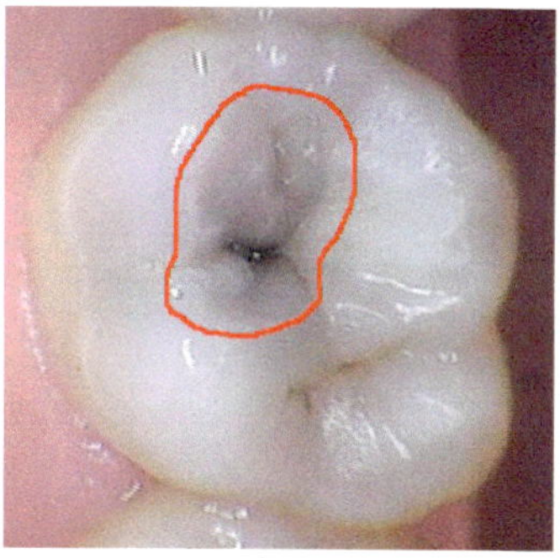

Deep occlusal caries in 16 as outlined.

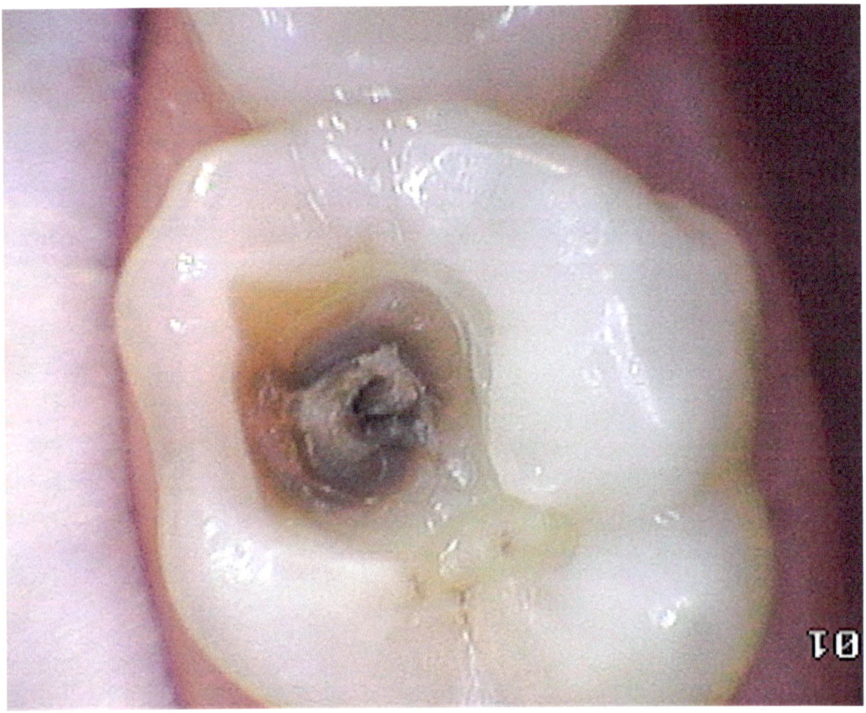


16 cavity almost caries-free.

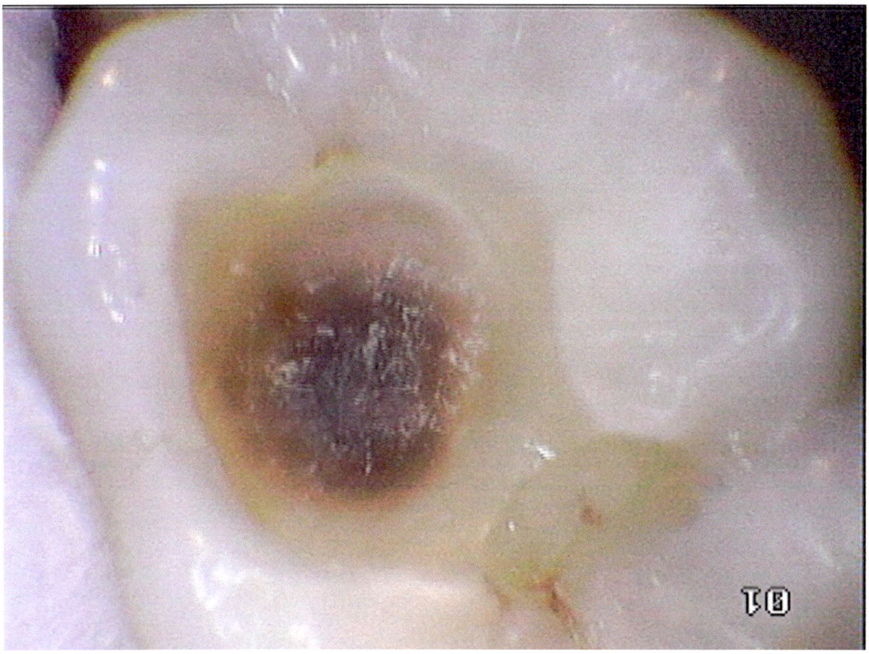

Affected but hard dentine remains at the base of the cavity. It is ready to restore.

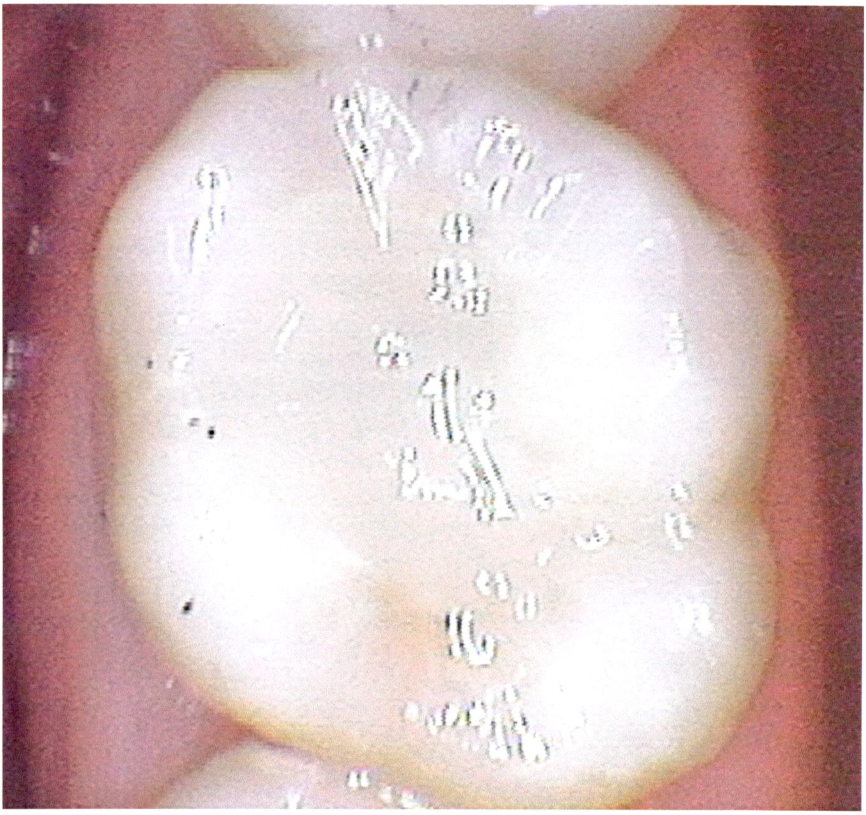

# *Interproximal* CARIES

This page and the next two pages.

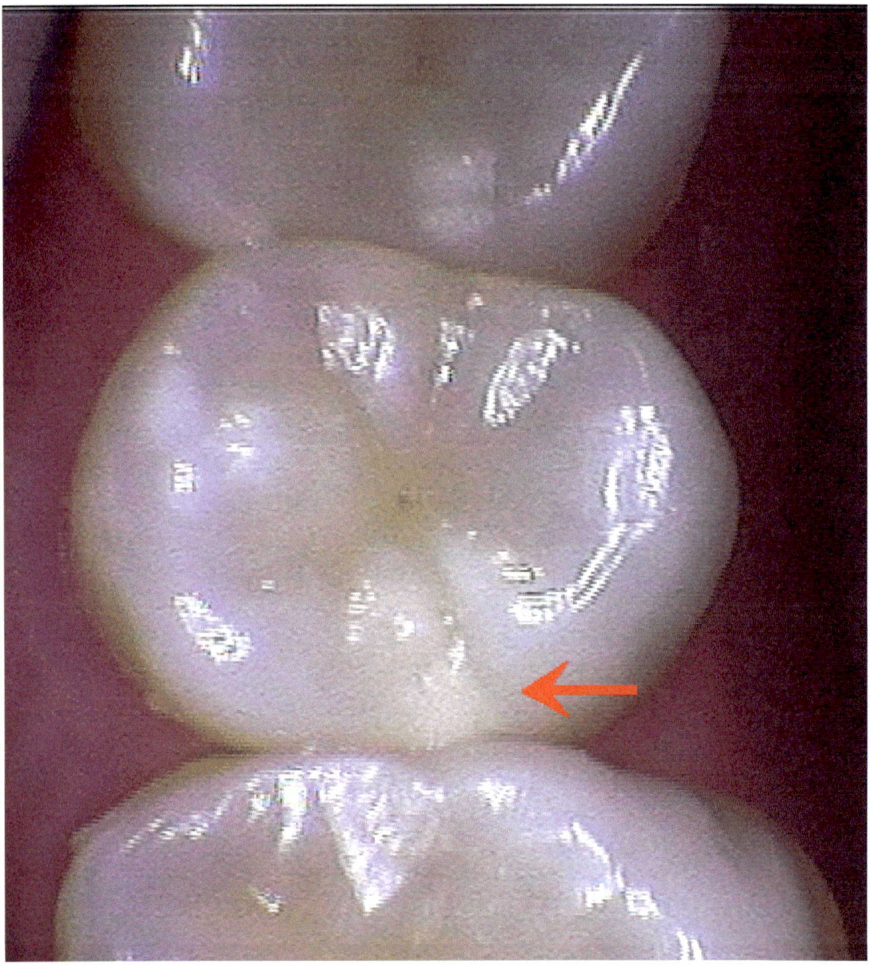

**ALWAYS** ensure that you dry the teeth so as to detect the subtle changes in tooth colour that occur, indicative of enamel decalcification and also of dentinal involvement, in this case tooth 15D.

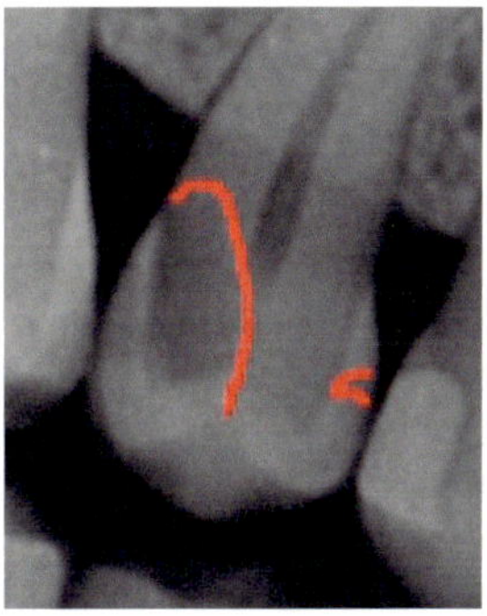

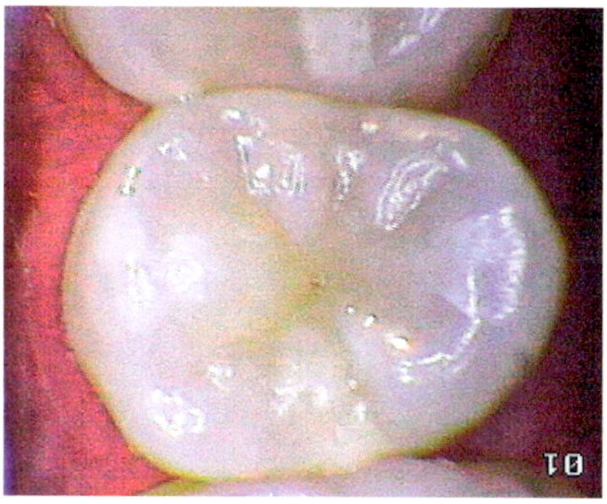

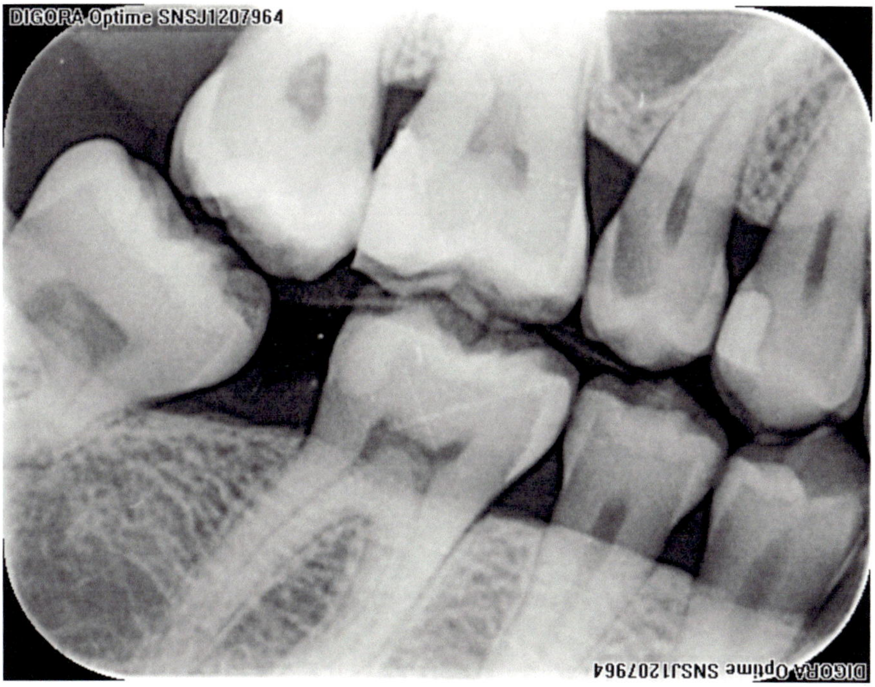


Had you not clinically seen the lesion in 15D, and not taken this bitewing x-ray, you would have missed a very deep cavity.

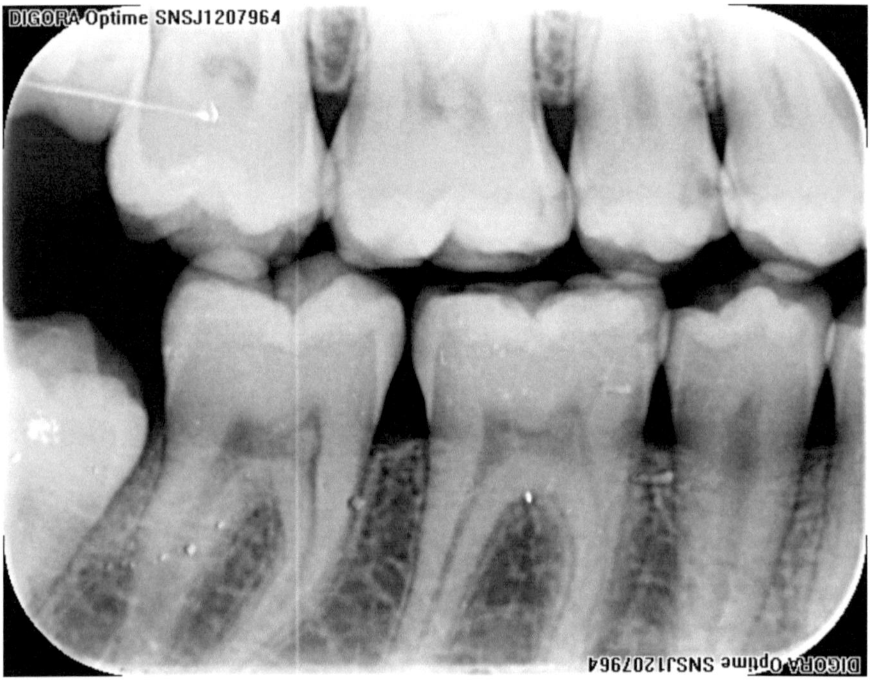


Many interstitial lesions are through the enamel and into the dentine.

Lesions in enamel only – to watch: 17M, 16D, 46D, 46M, 47M.
Caries just into dentine – to clean and fill: 16M, 15D, 14D.
Deeper caries with more dentine involvement: 15M.

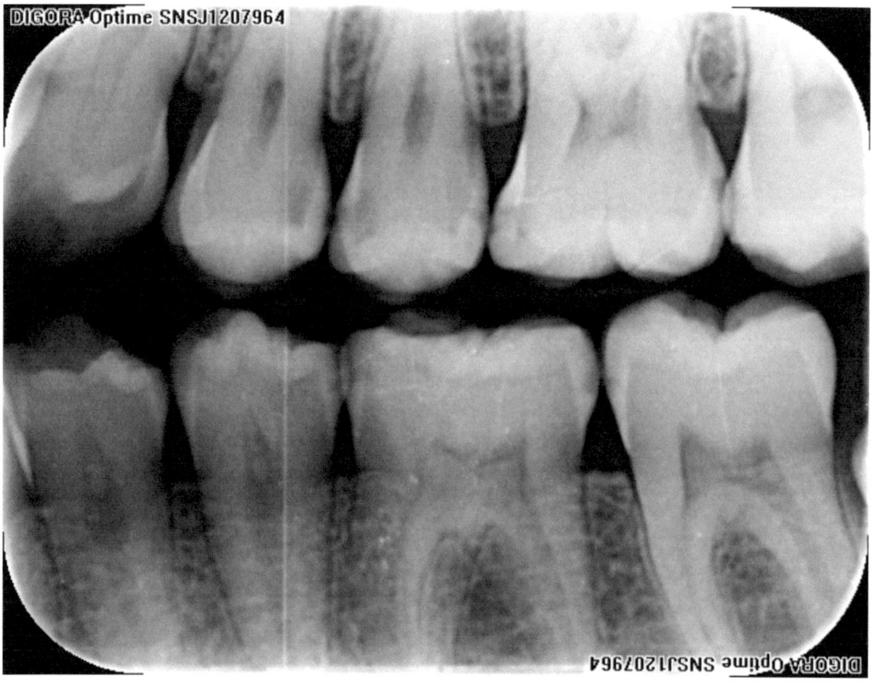


Lesions in enamel only – to watch: 25D, 26D, 36D, 37M, 35D.
Lesions just into dentine: 36M, 26M
Resin Infiltration? Fluoride?
Deeper caries with more dentine involvement: 24D, 25M.

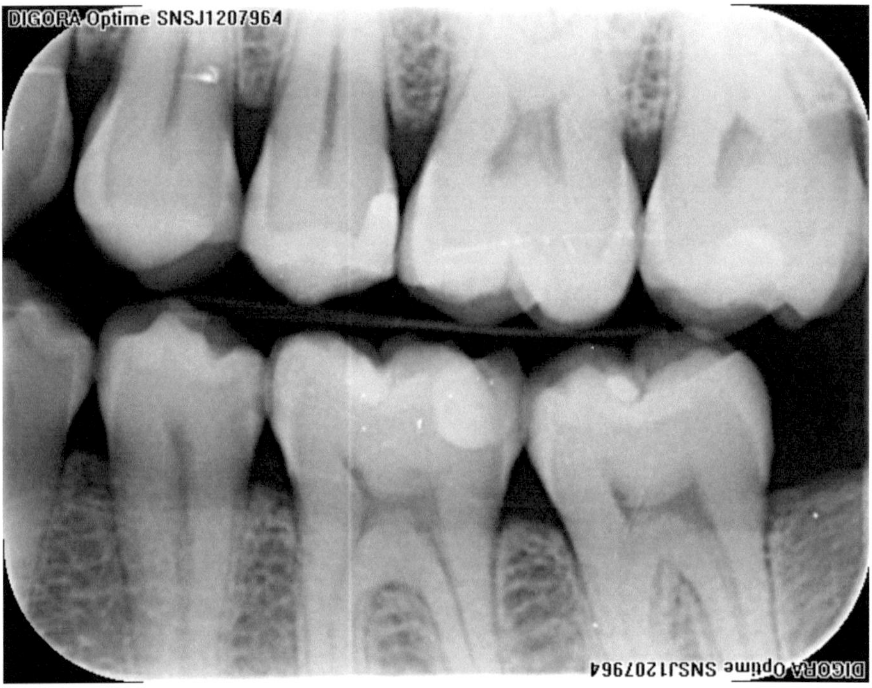


There are enamel lesions in 23D, 24D, 25M, 26D, 27M, 36M+D. In 35D the lesion has almost reached the enamel/dentine junction. Motivate this patient to optimise their oral hygiene including the regular use of floss. You will need to monitor the teeth over time, with bitewing radiographs taken again 12-18 months later.

This page and the next four pages.

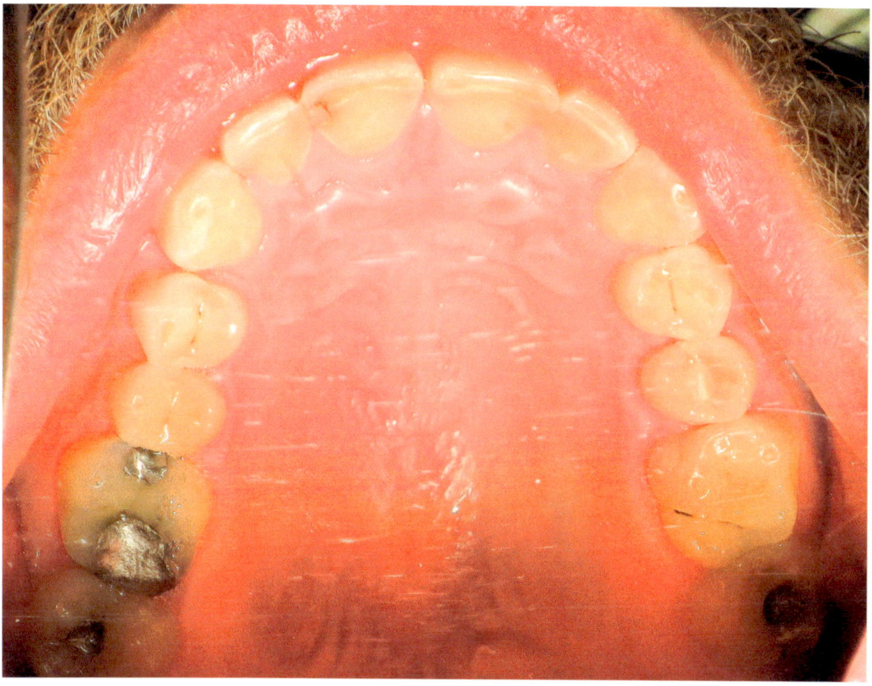

I want you to search for caries around an existing filling, and enamel changes where two other  teeth touch each other.

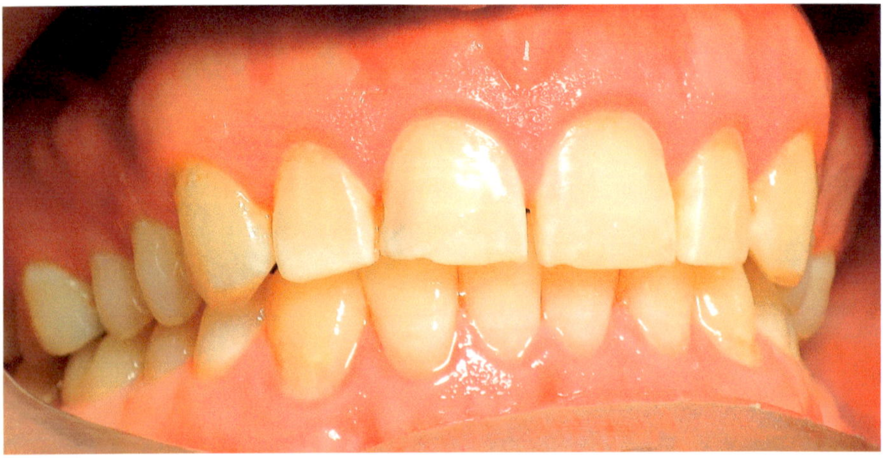

Can you see caries anywhere?

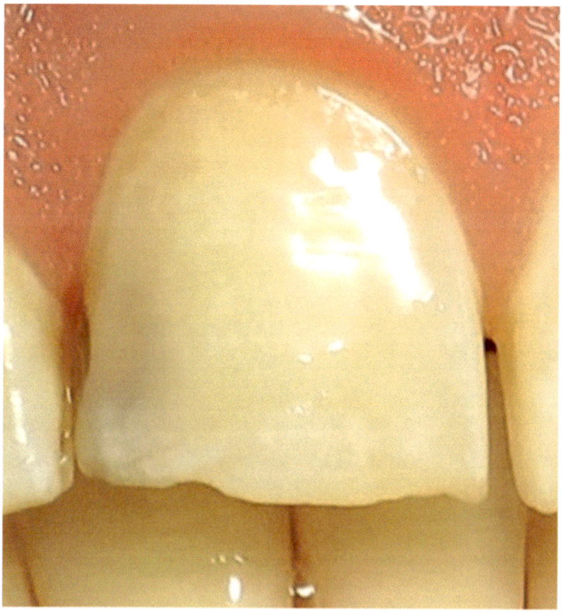

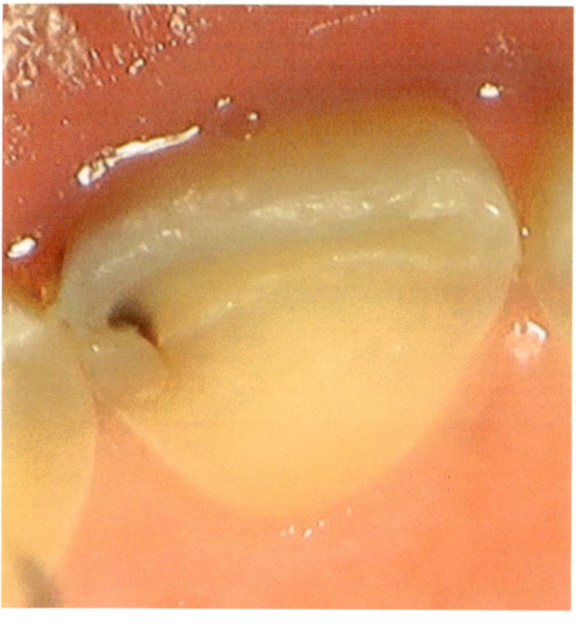

11 has a distal-palatal composite filling with caries around it. The caries will have arisen due to leakage around the filling.

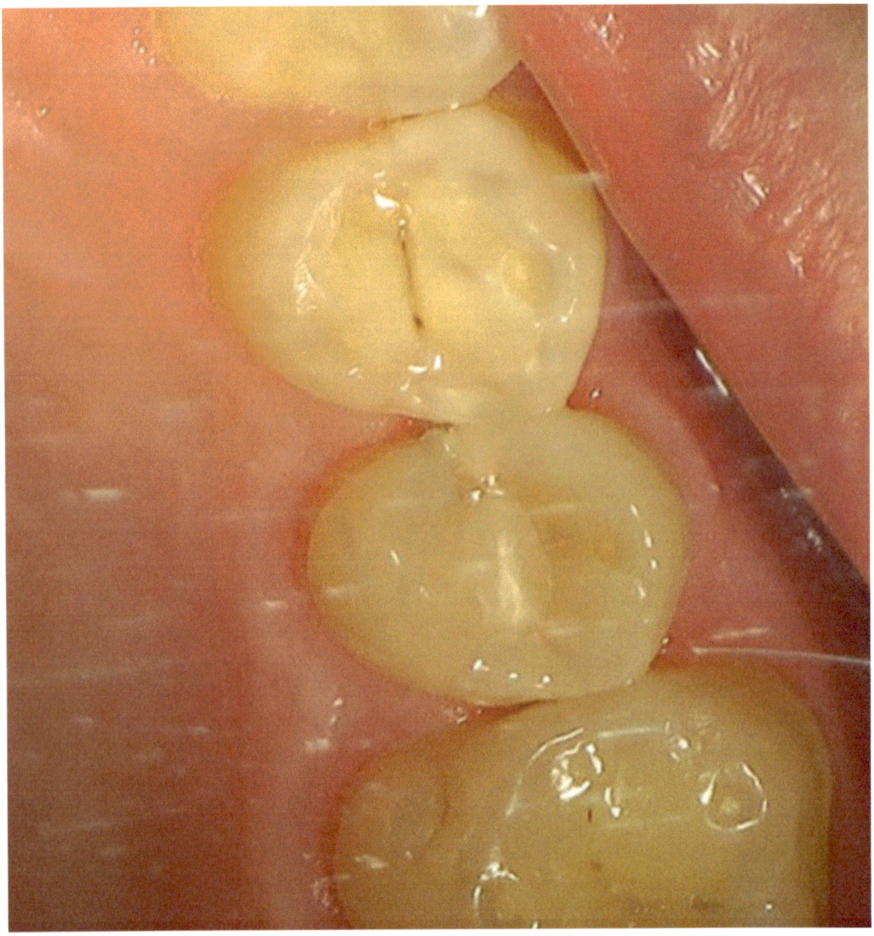

Look carefully at 24D and 25M. See the subtle colour changes? There is decalcification on 24D that appears to be restricted to the enamel only, and with that in 25M appearing to have spread into the dentine.

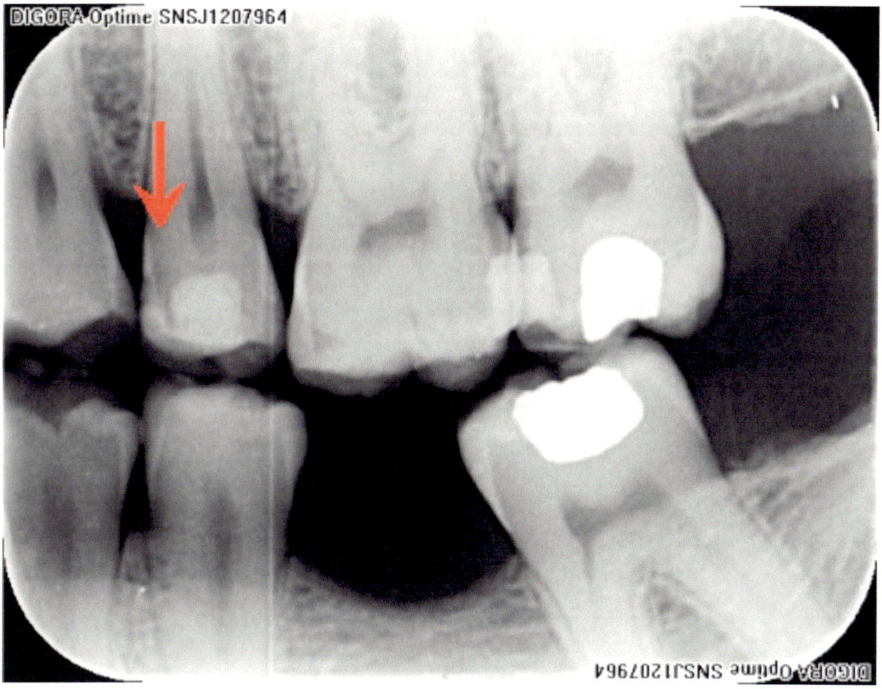


25 requires an MO filling due to caries spreading in the dentine. 24D has a lesion restricted to enamel only – to watch.

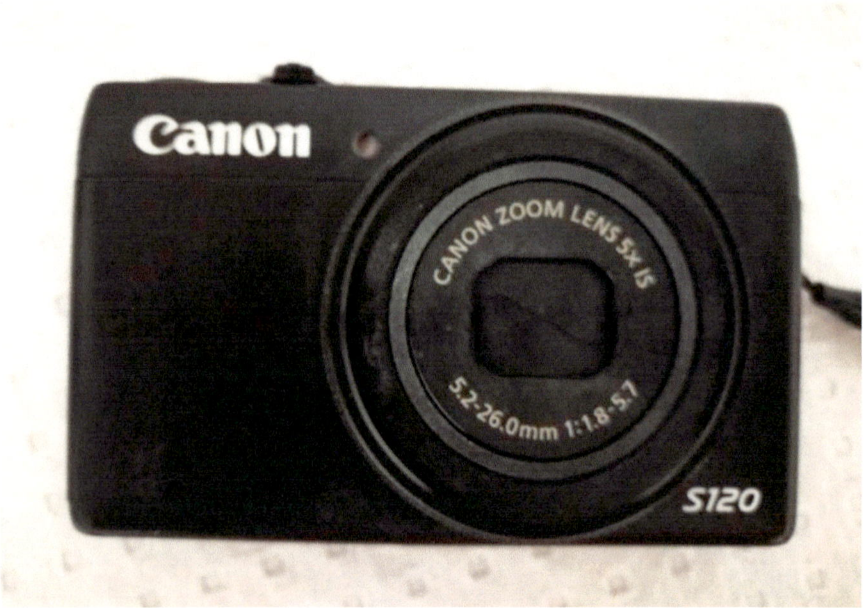


Camera used for photographs.

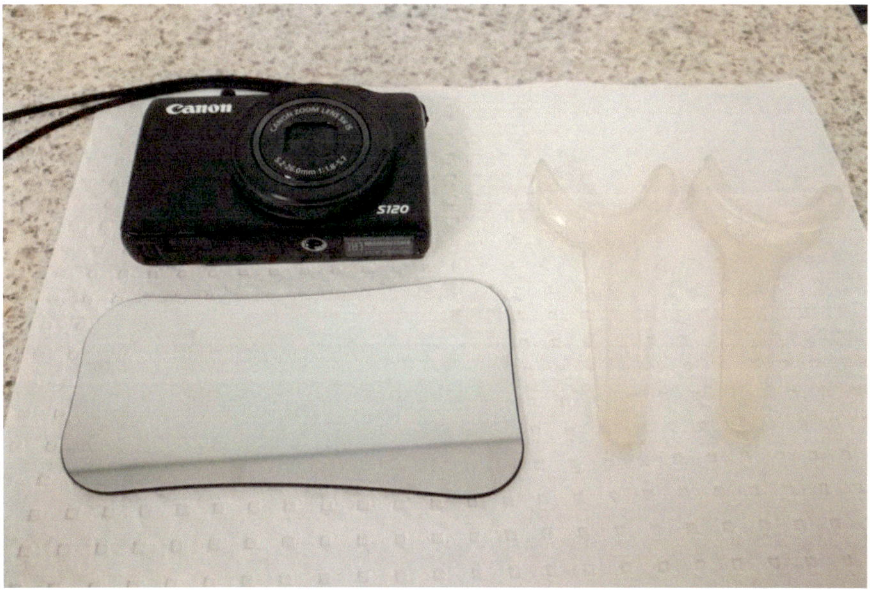


Camera, lip retractors and mirror.

# Bitewing radiographs

Bitewing radiographs are extremely useful to see how things are where teeth touch each other, i.e. interproximal surfaces, and also to see how things are beneath existing restorations.

For them to be diagnostically useful you must standardise the way that you take the radiographs, in three dimensions. Firstly, have the patient's occlusal plane parallel to the floor. Secondly, have the x-ray tube on a 10° downward shift. Thirdly, ensure that the tube is placed at a 90° angle to the line of the arch, in other words perpendicular to the contact points.

In this way you will obtain diagnostically useful bitewing radiographs. The advantage of standardising the way you take EVERY bitewing radiograph is that you can then track and monitor and compare with subsequent radiographs over years and decades.

Early enamel lesions can then be compared and tracked, as can be areas of small radiolucency beneath old fillings that you opt to monitor.

Three examples follow of the benefit of taking bitewing x-rays consistently the same way every time.

August 2015

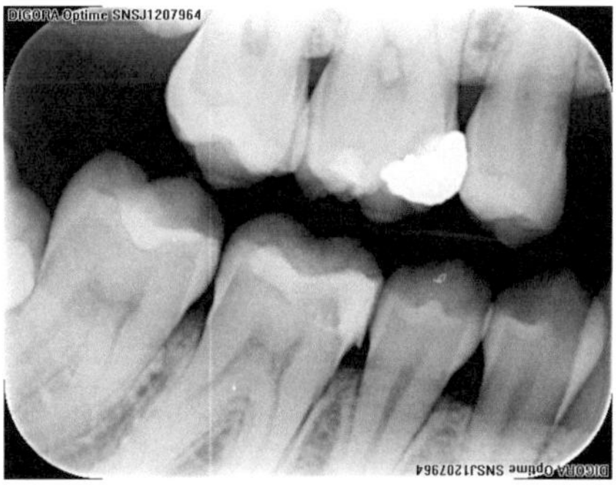


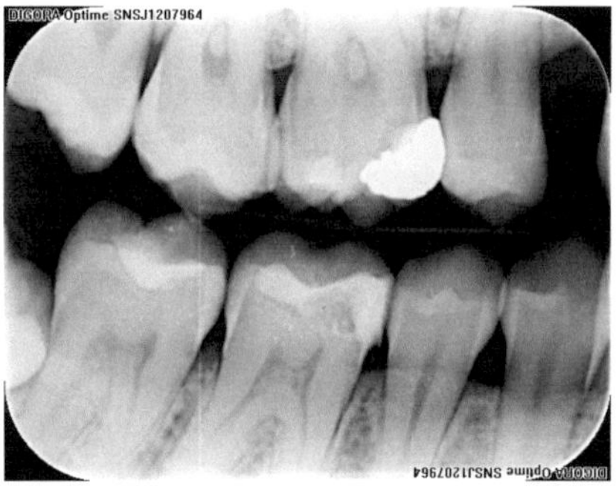


July 2017

Bitewing x-rays taken two years apart, taken in such a way that true comparisons can be made. We are tracking 16MO, 25DO, 26MO, 27O, 36MO, and 46MO. There have been no changes in two years. This interesting case is discussed in more detail on pages 174-180.

April 2015

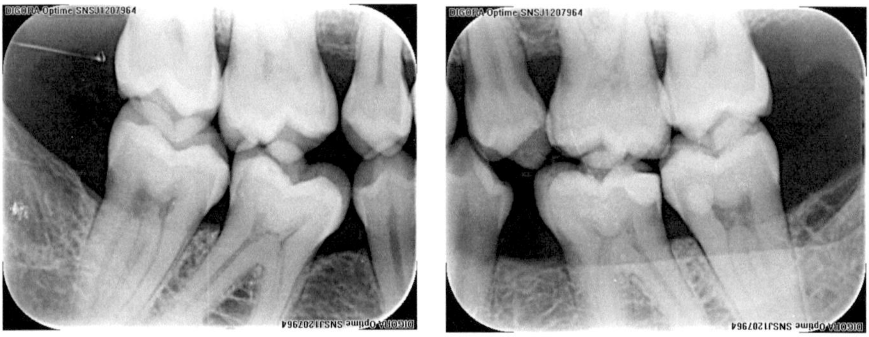


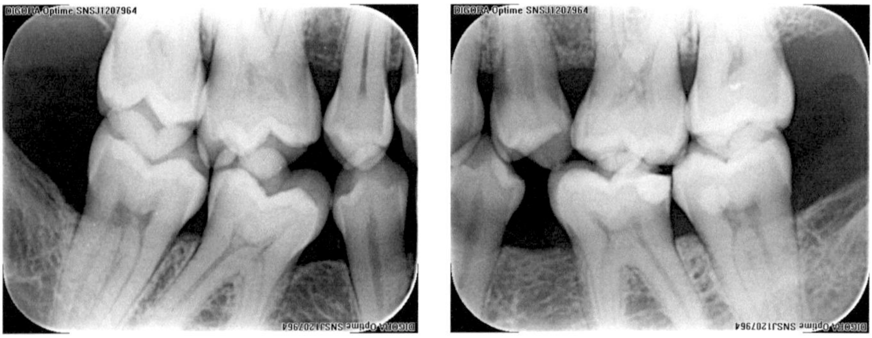


November 2018

Consistency in taking bitewing radiographs allows you to check on areas you opted to monitor. They are very useful for checking on alveolar crestal bone levels too.

September 2013

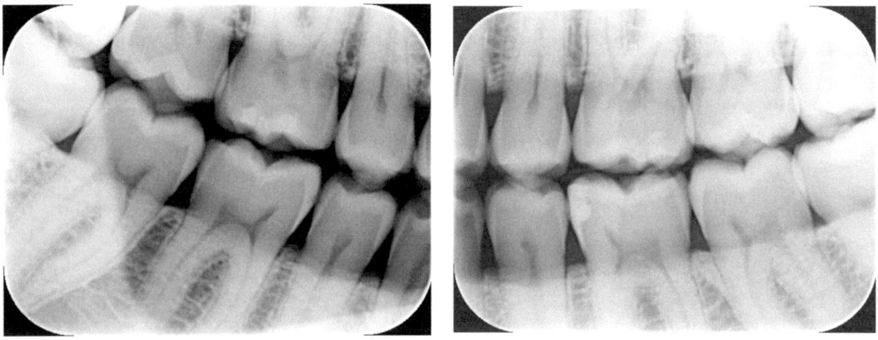

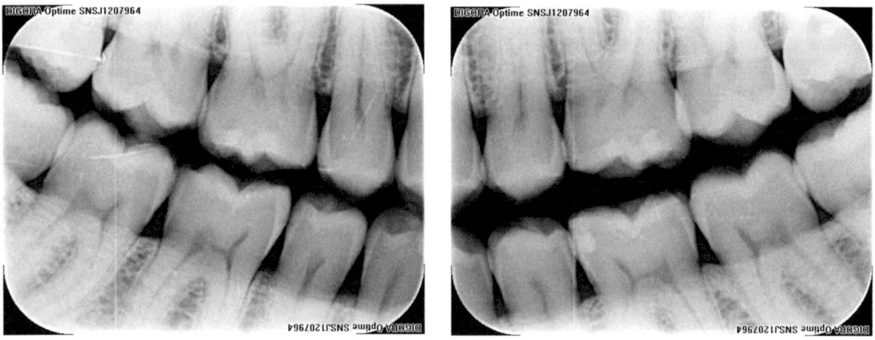


February 2017

With these x-rays you have to look very closely to discern that one set is not a copy of the other. This must be your aim with bitewing radiographs in particular.

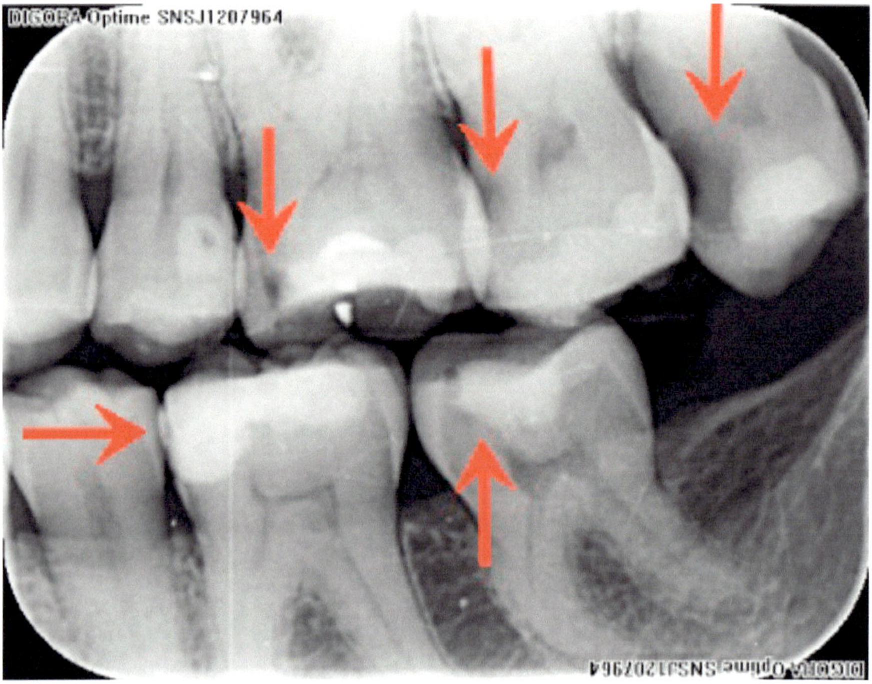


This patient presented saying toothache from 36. 28 was the main problem. There is caries in 26M and 27M, and the fillings in 26O, 36MO and 37O need to be assessed clinically.

The patient could not feel the cavity in 28M as tooth structure had not broken down buccally, palatally or occlusally.

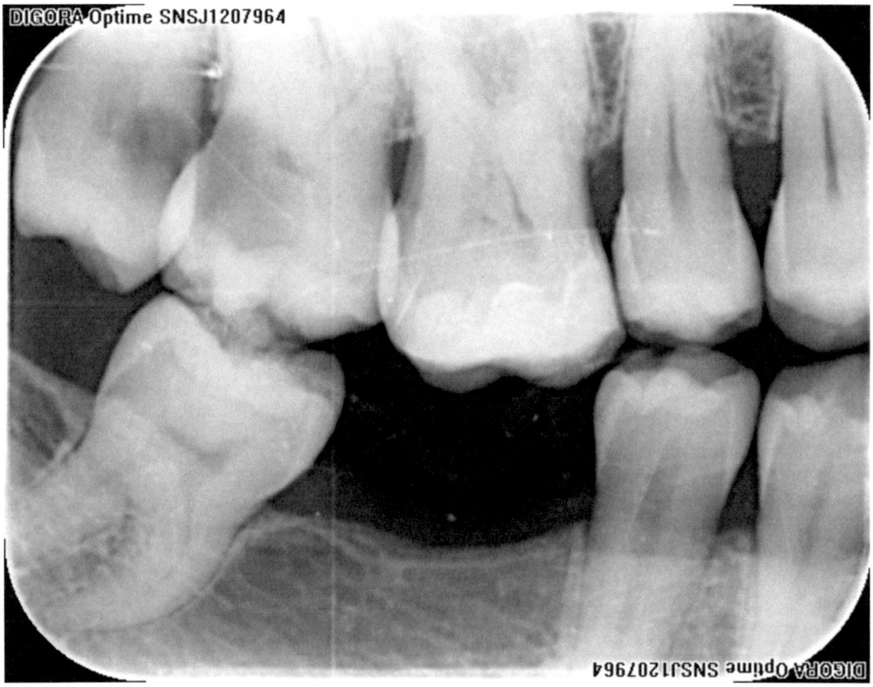


The same patient, she never returned for 17 and 18, until the 17 broke five months later and toothache forced her to seek treatment.

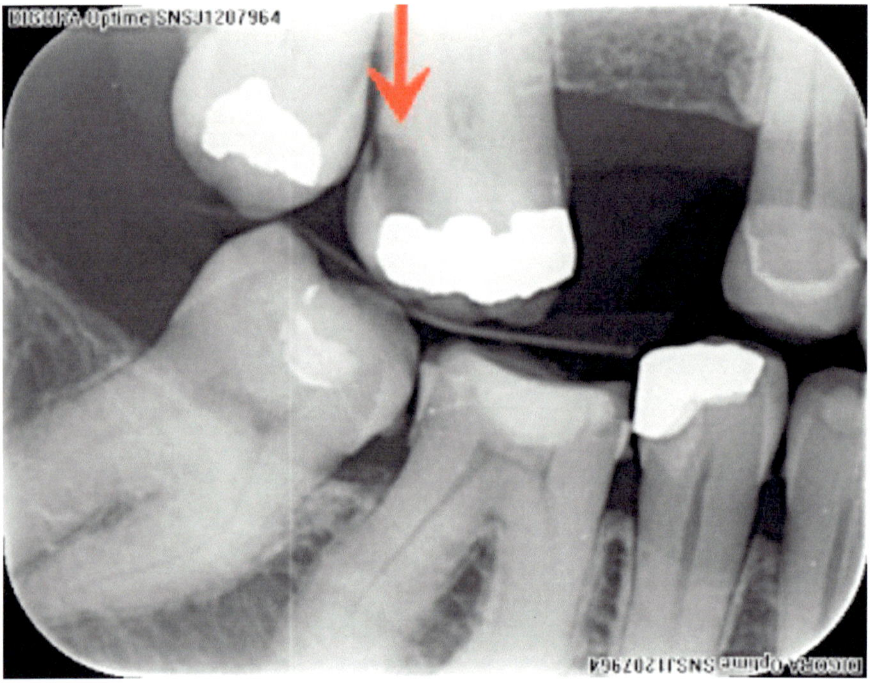


When you see caries this deep (17D) and knowing that the extent of the decay is greater than what the x-ray shows, advise the patient of the possibility that the caries could be reaching the pulp. Have there been any symptoms suggestive of a pulpitis?

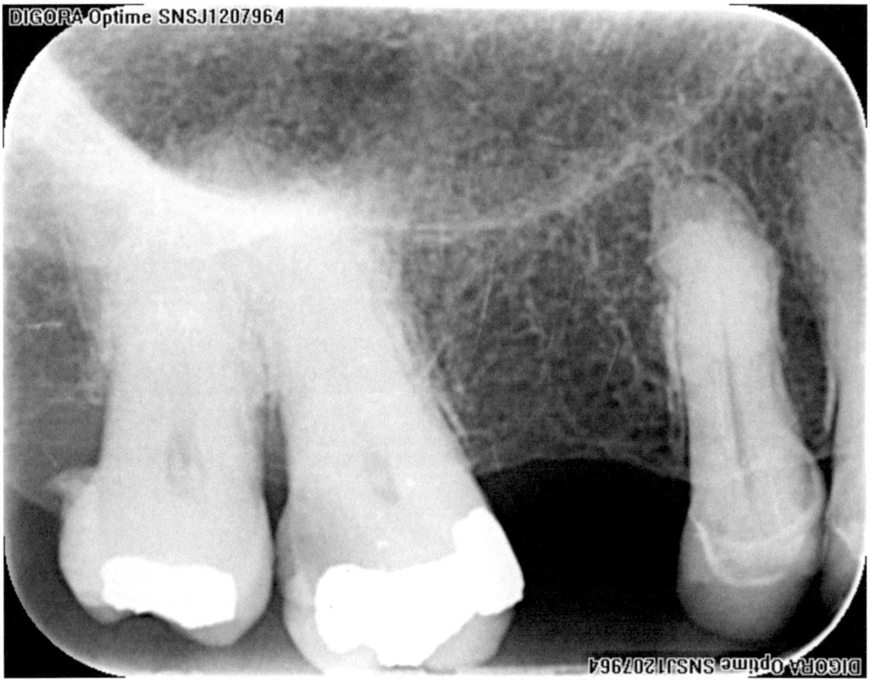


I took a periapical radiograph as well to see if there was any periapical pathology.

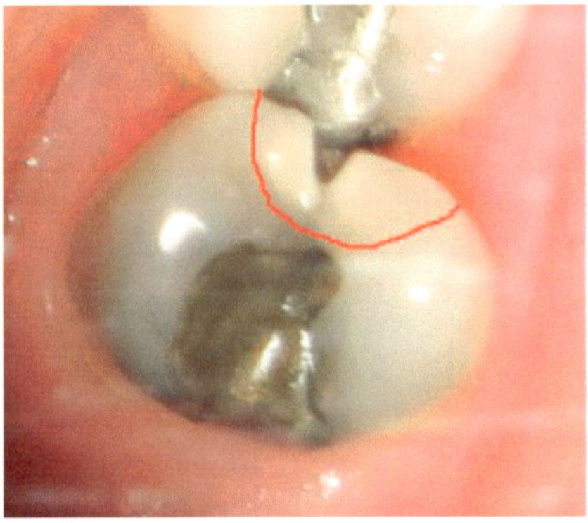

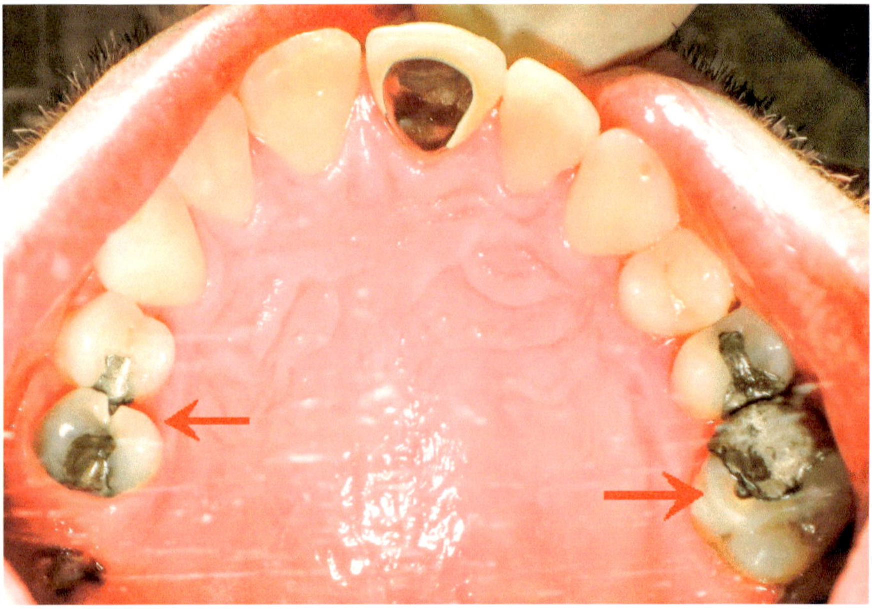

Breakdown 15M. The creamy-yellow colour changes indicate the caries is wide and deep.

See the occlusal caries palatal to the amalgam filling in 26? Clinical and radiographic correlation will indicate whether you replace the entire amalgam filling in 26 or whether you work locally if the caries is not widespread or extensive.

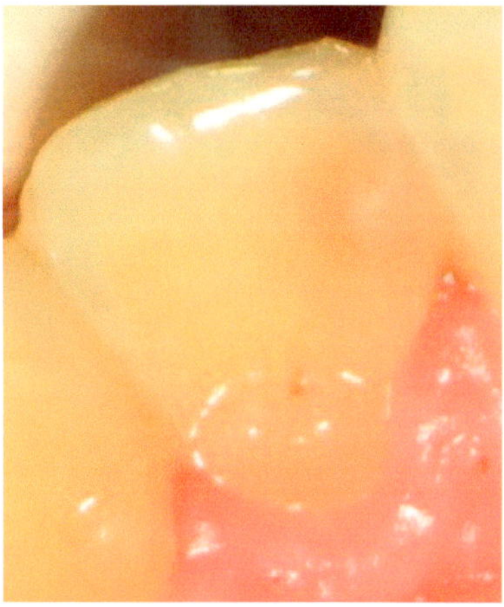

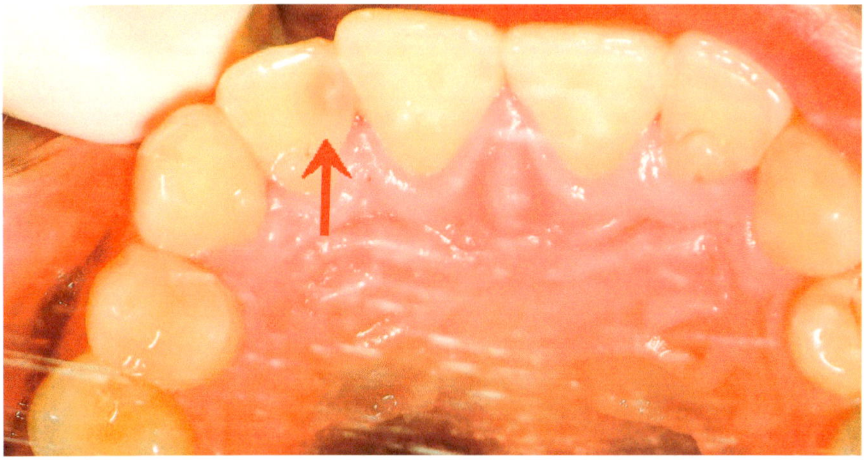

There is enamel and dentine involvement in 12MP region.

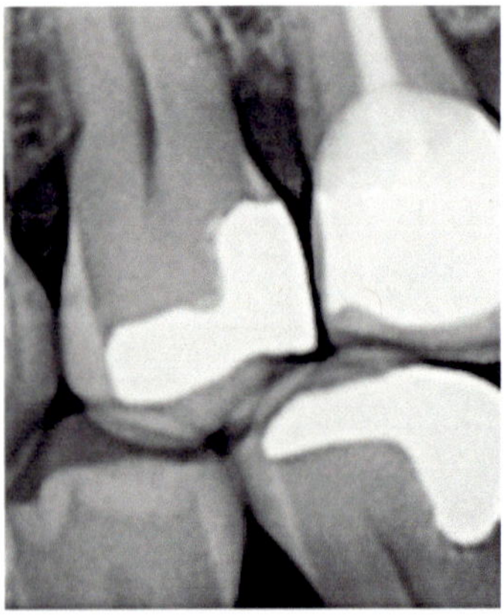

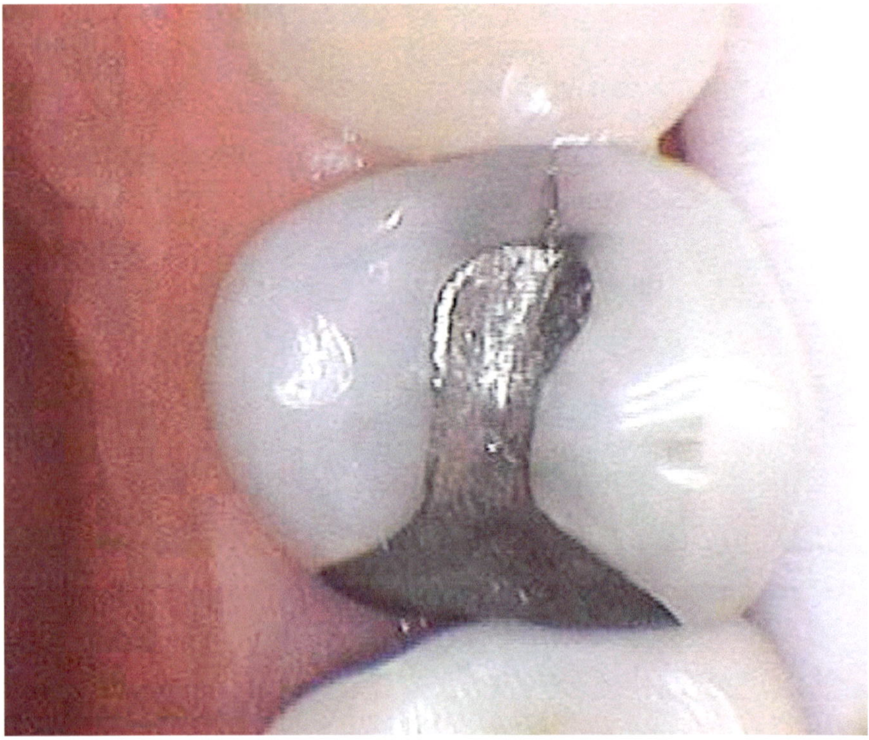

There is a crack in 24 mesial marginal ridge and caries spreading at the enamel-dentine junction.

This page and the next four pages.

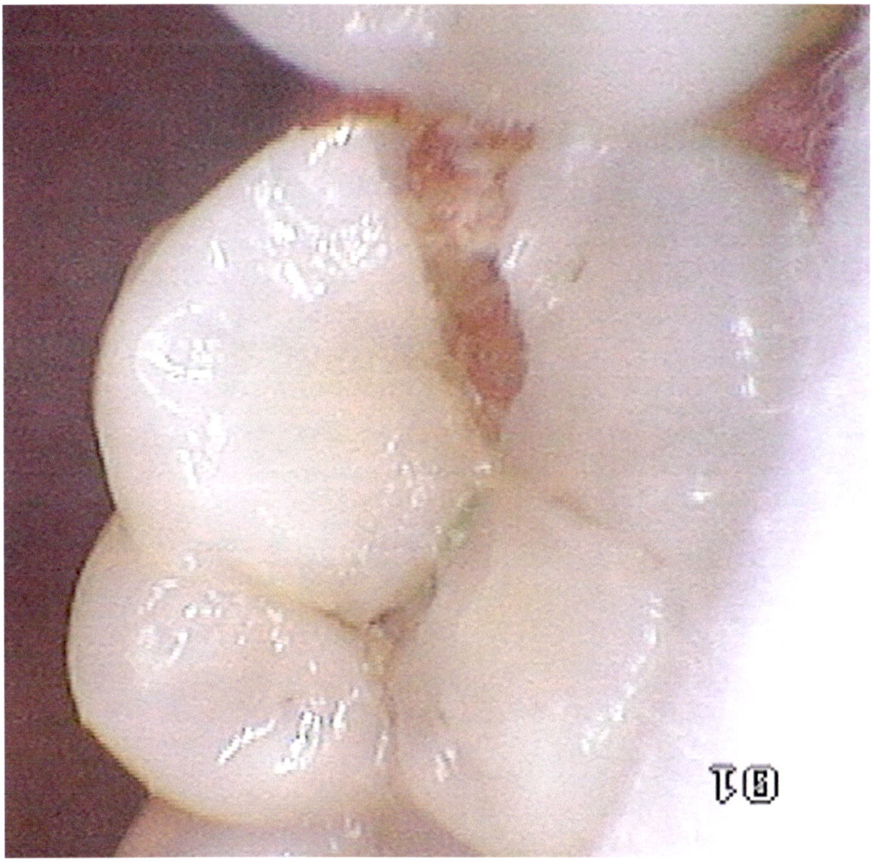

Experience will tell you once you see this cavity that the caries is very deep. There may be pulpal involvement. What are the signs and symptoms? There may be a mesial → distal sagittal fracture.

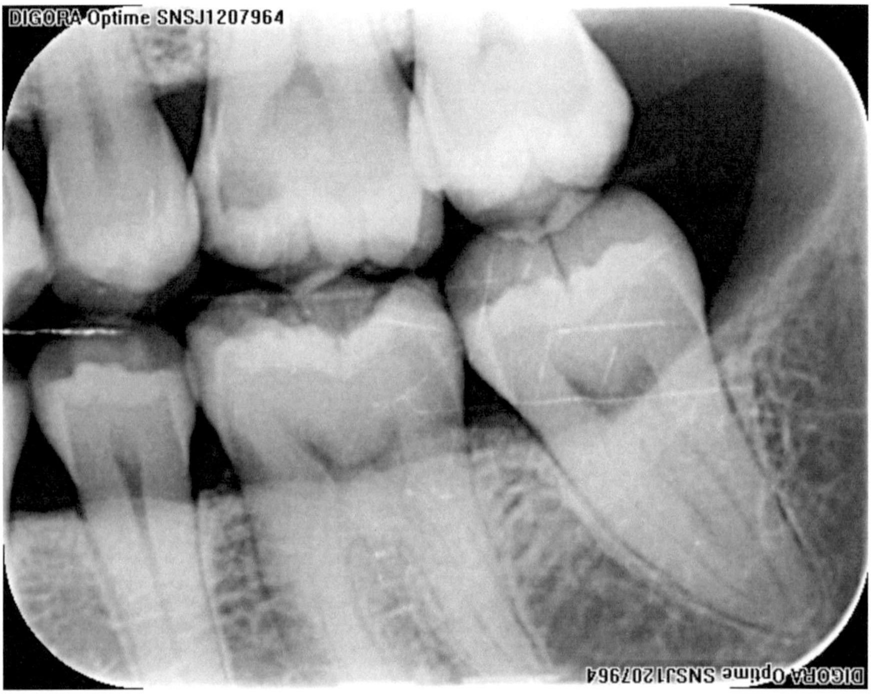


You must caution the patient of the high probability of a carious exposure before you commence treatment.

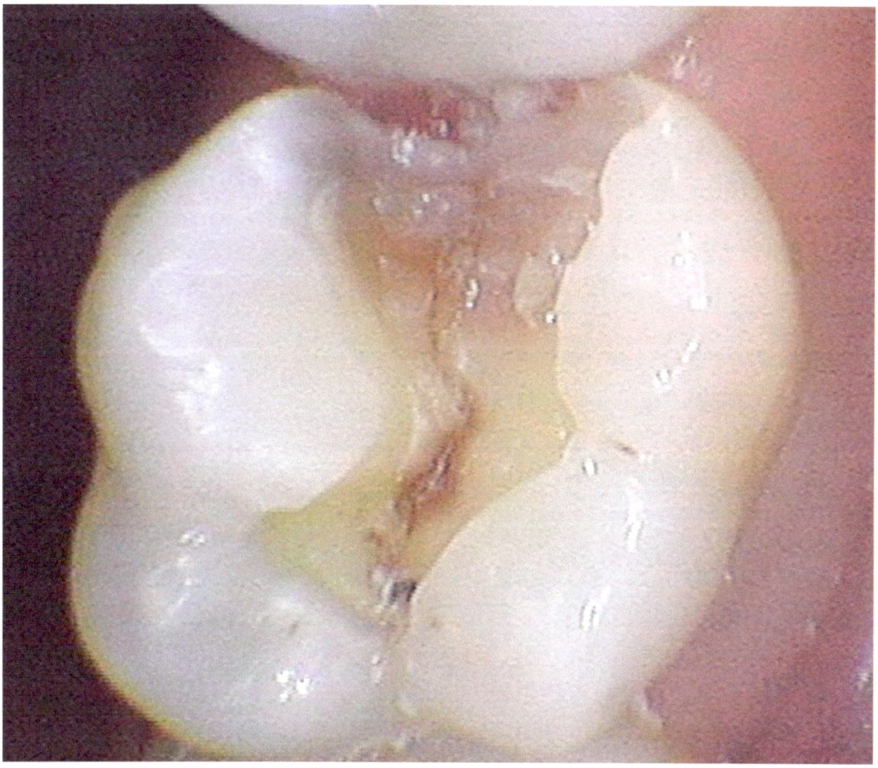

Caries still present mesially. Note that creamy, light caries is the rapidly spreading form of caries.

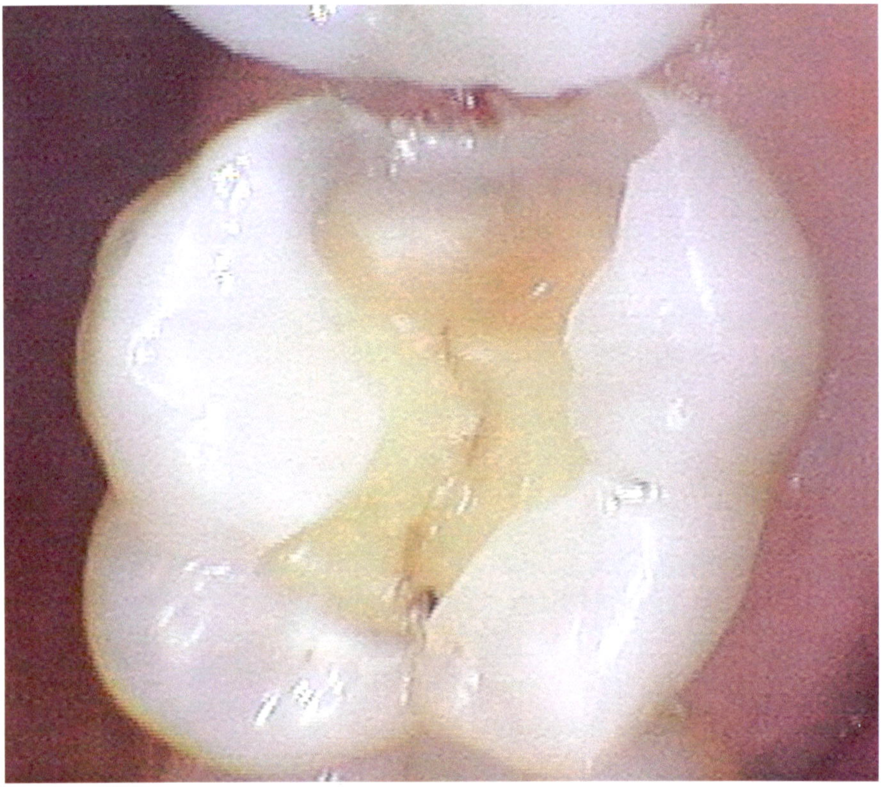

Advise the patient that there is a crack in the floor of the cavity and that the tooth may require a crown.

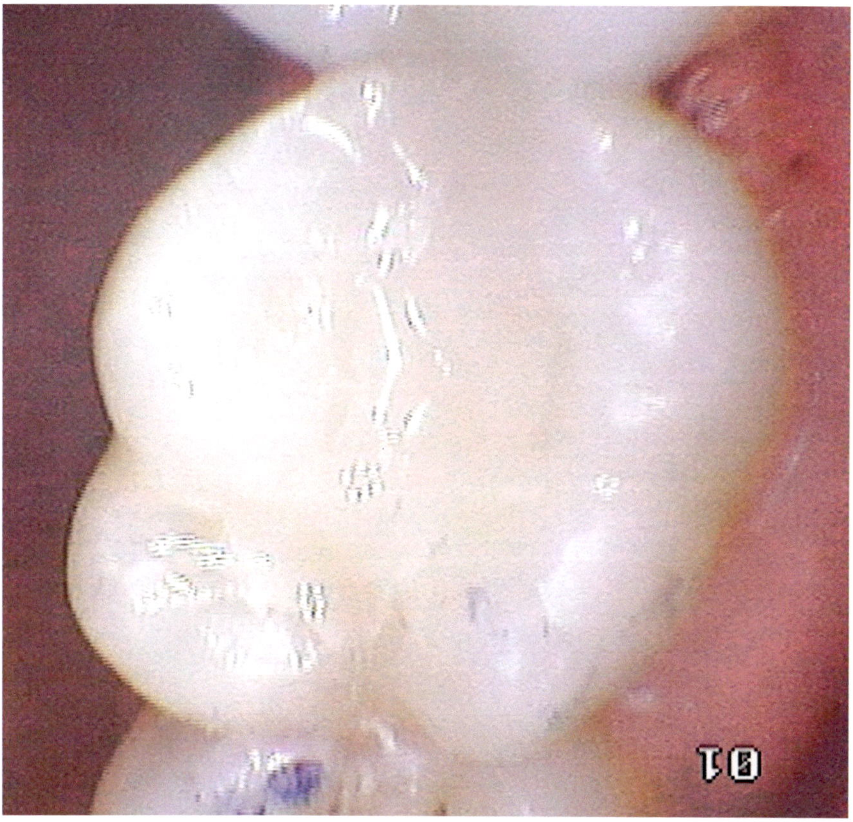

Ask the patient to contact you if he gets any symptoms on chewing. Due to the crack in the tooth, a crown may be required.

These are NOT good bitewing radiographs. Diagnostically they tell you very little. The patient has not closed enough on the film holder, resulting in you not being able to assess 17, 27, 36, 37, 44, 45, 46 and 47.

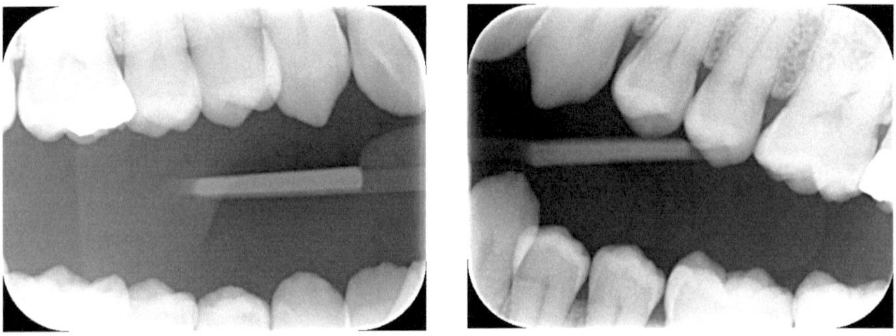

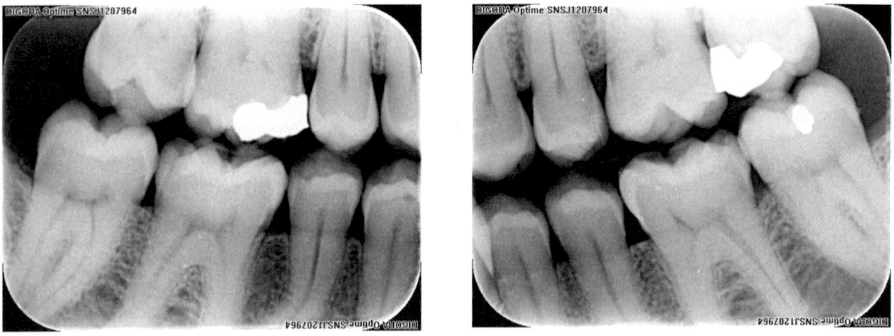


These are good bitewing radiographs – of the same patient. These radiographs have been taken with the patient biting on a thin tab (hence the term "bitewing"), allowing the teeth to come together easily, revealing all the coronal parts of the teeth and the alveolar crestal bone.

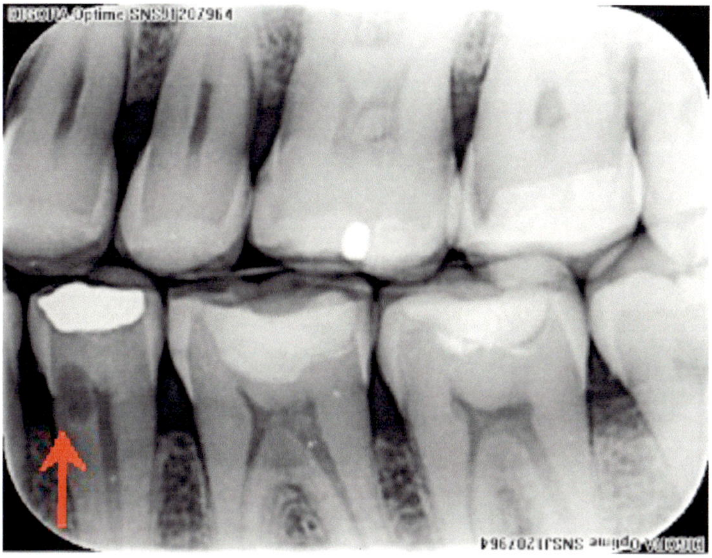


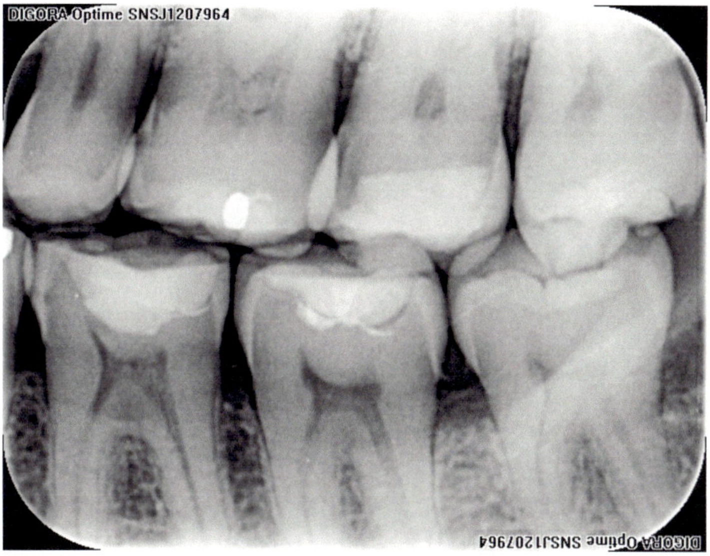


Sometimes there is a need to take two bitewing radiographs on each side if the length/span of the arch is long. On the lower bitewing you can see all of the third molars, but not enough of the premolars, and the large problem in 35MB would not be seen radiographically unless this second bitewing (upper one) was taken, placed more anteriorly.

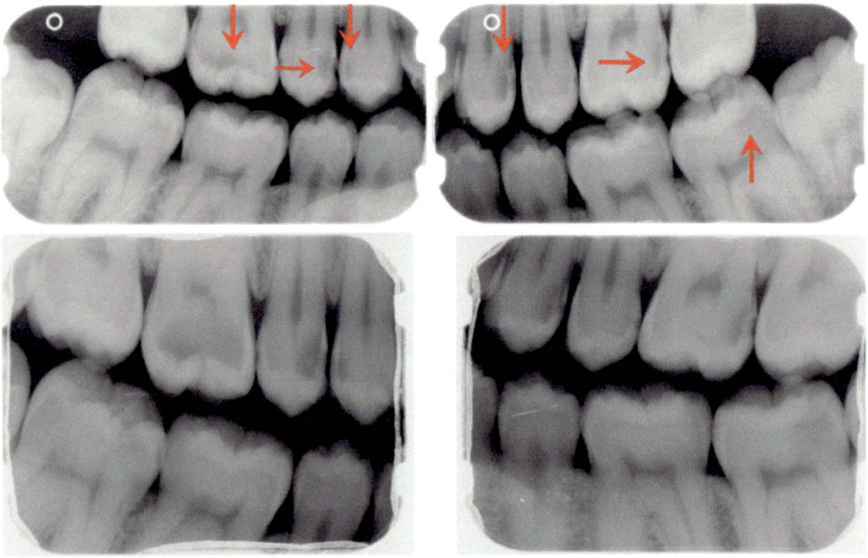

Top bitewings – patient age 16, told of at least 6 cavities. Patient and parents counselled on the importance of attending to the caries and that the sooner this done the better. He could not feel the cavities and did not return for them to be attended to.

Lower bitewings – patient now age 19, presented with pain from 16, which now had extensive caries and had broken. You can see that the caries in 16O, 15M, 14D, 24D, 26D and 37O is now much deeper.

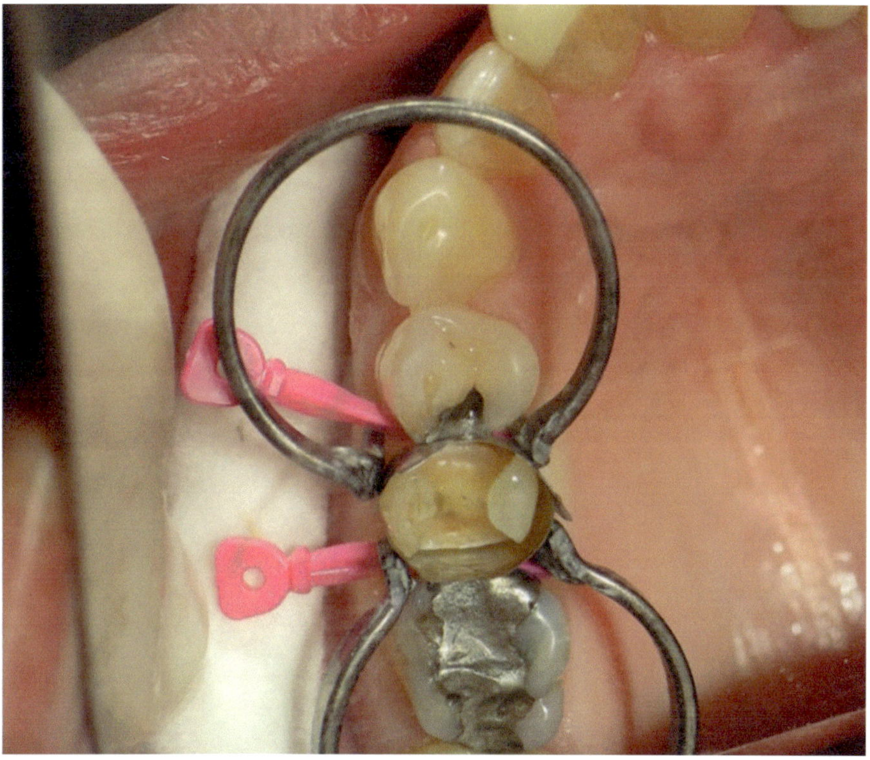

The use of sectional matrices allows you to achieve excellent, well shaped contour and tight contacts.

This page and the next two pages.

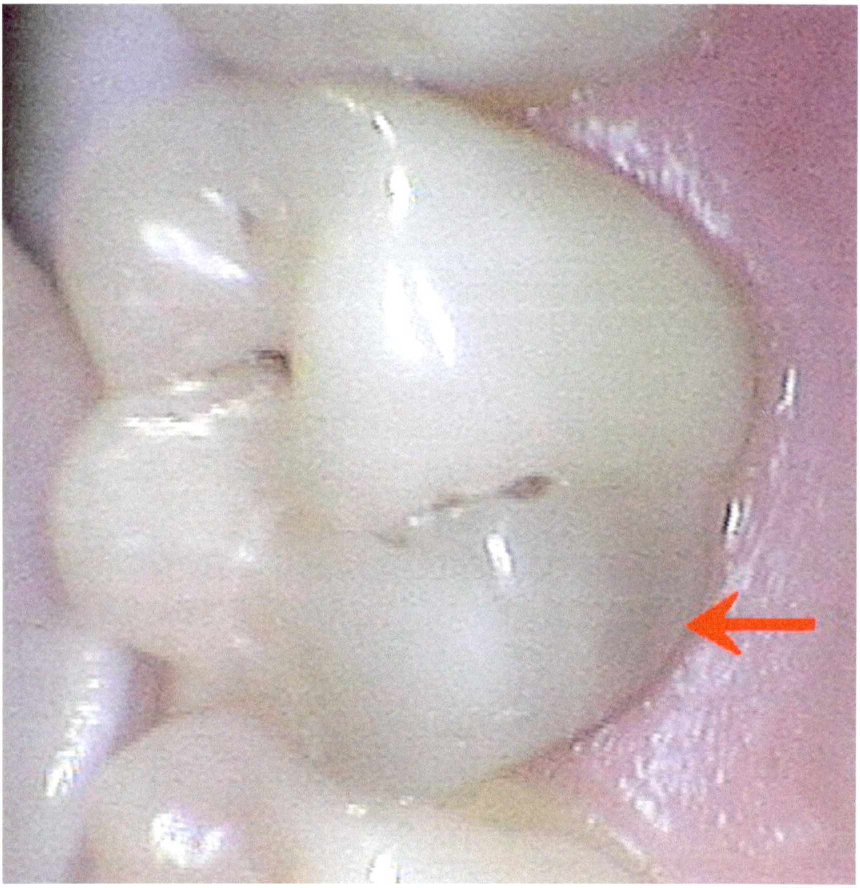

Caries around and beneath an existing 16DO filling.

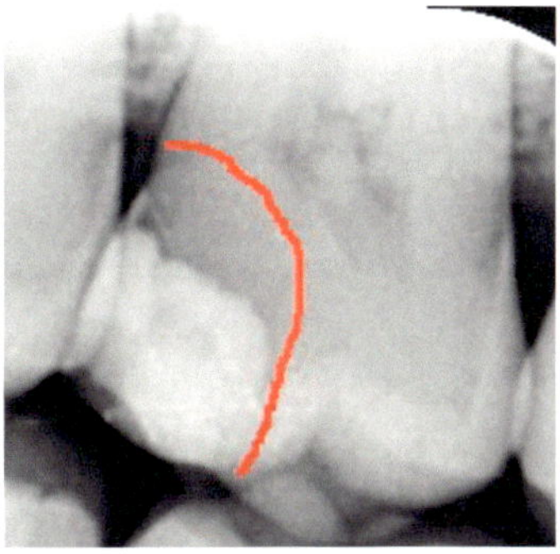

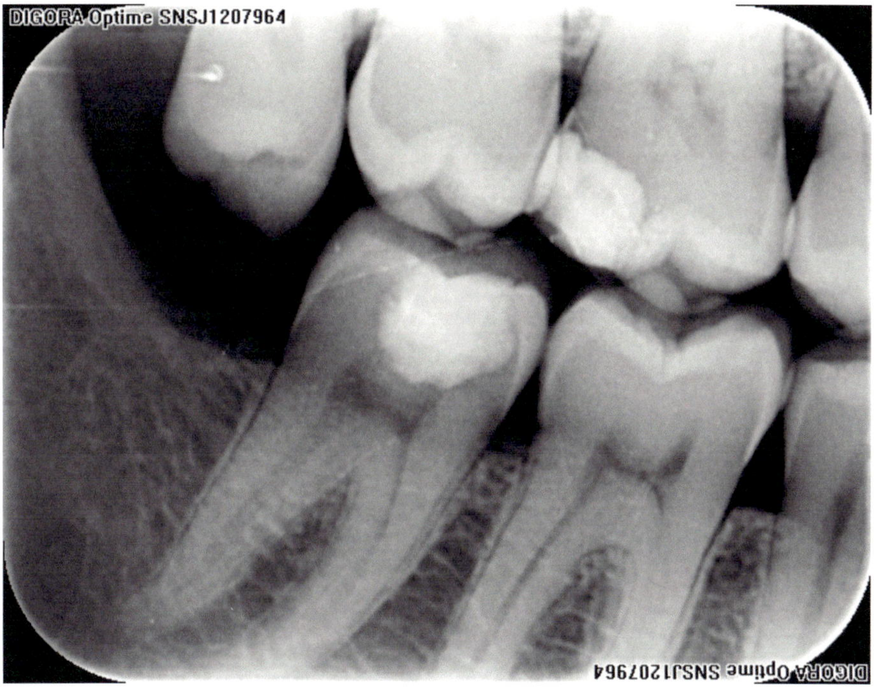


A right bitewing x-ray confirms 16DOP caries is very deep and there may be pulpal involvement. The patient has no symptoms. Advise the patient that if the caries has reached the pulp that the tooth may need more than just a filling.

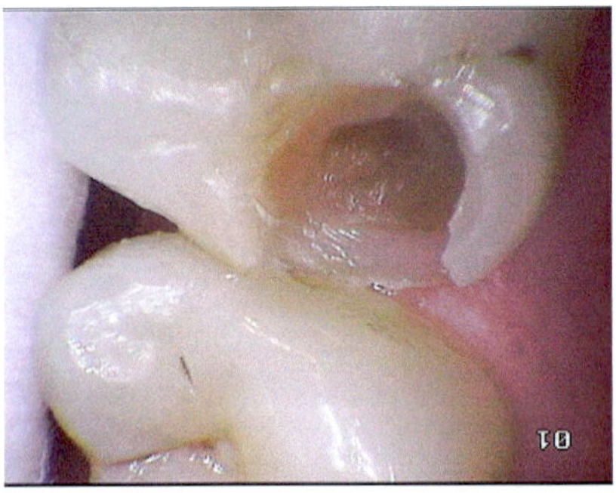

After removing the filling.

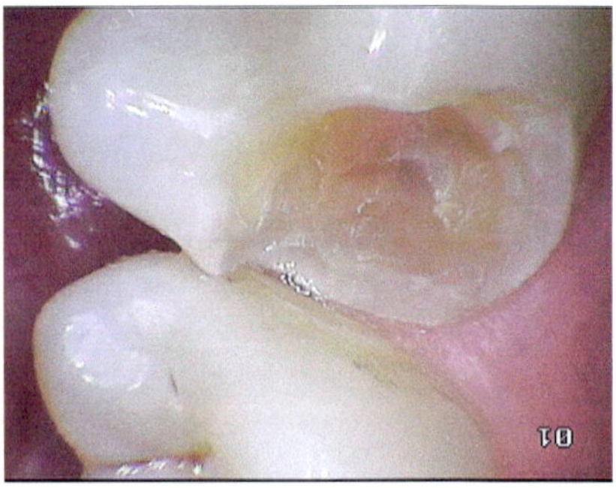

The cavity is partly clean.

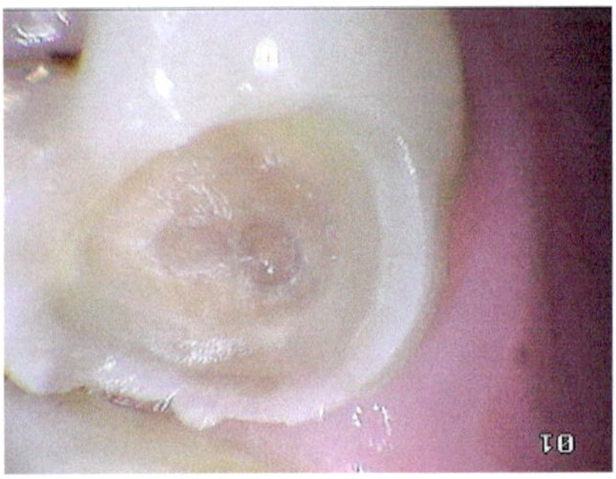

Caries-free. Note secondary dentine. Very deep but no exposure.

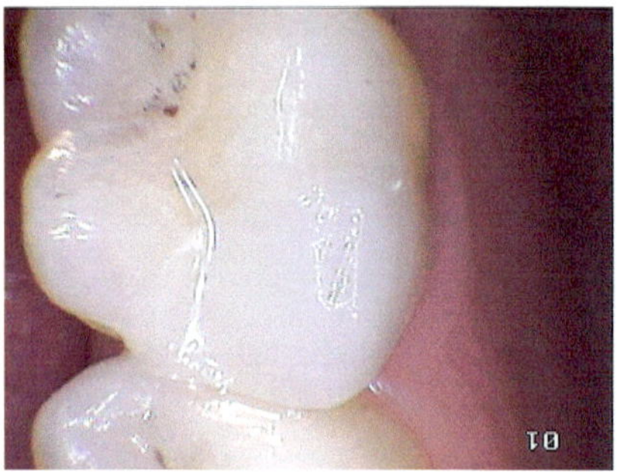

Cavity restored.

Depending on your restoration protocol, you may place a lining at the base of the cavity in the deepest area over the pulp.

This page and the next four pages.

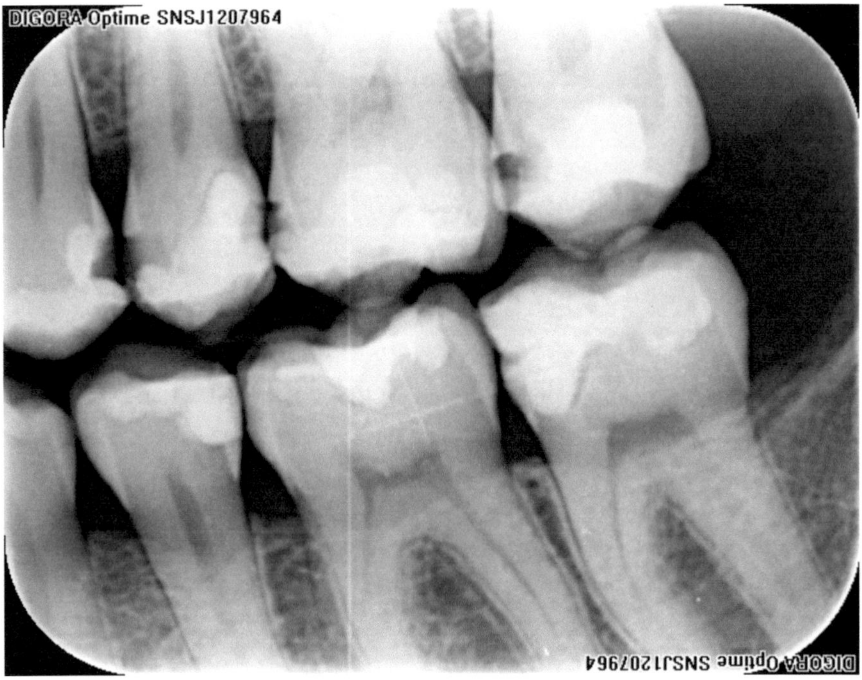


Cavities 24D, 25M+D, 26M, 27M, 37M(?) and 35D

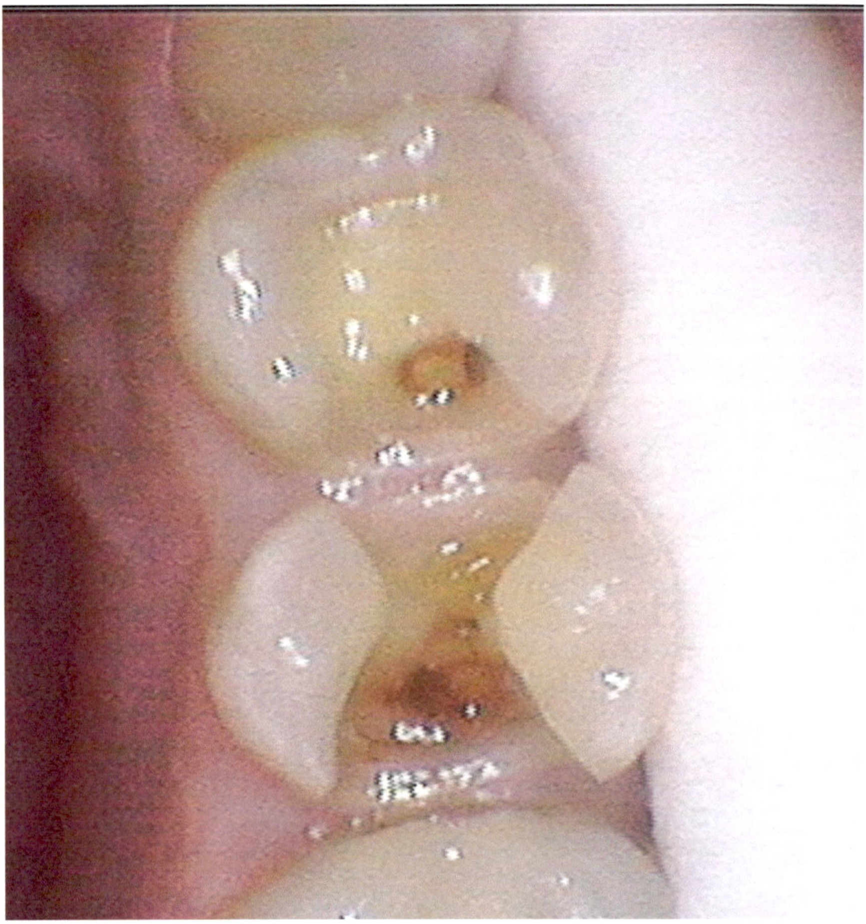

24 and 25 fillings removed, the cavities caries-free.

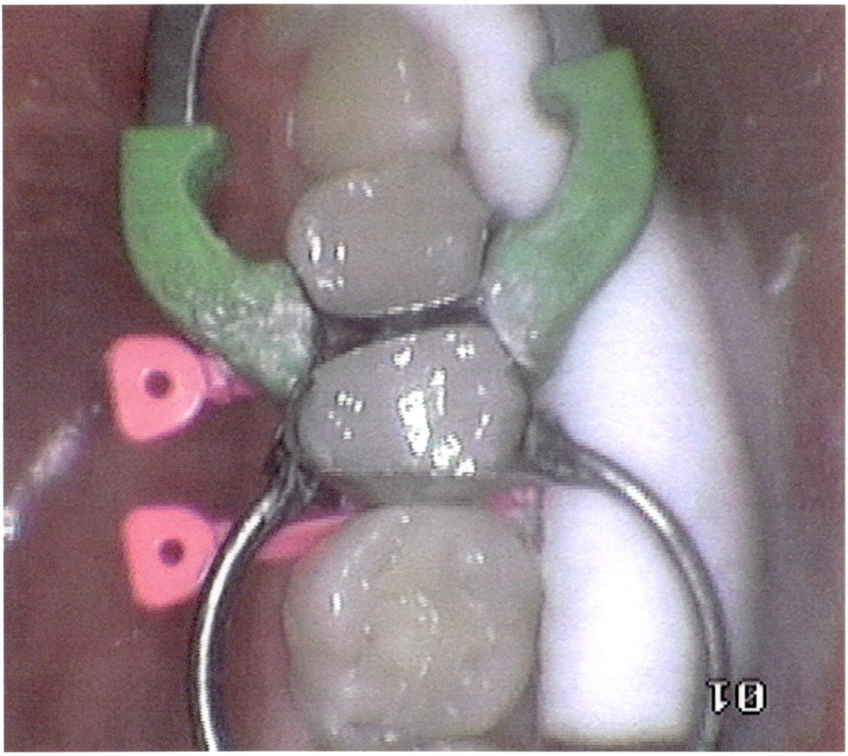

Palodent sectional matrices, Bitine ring, V-ring, wedges.

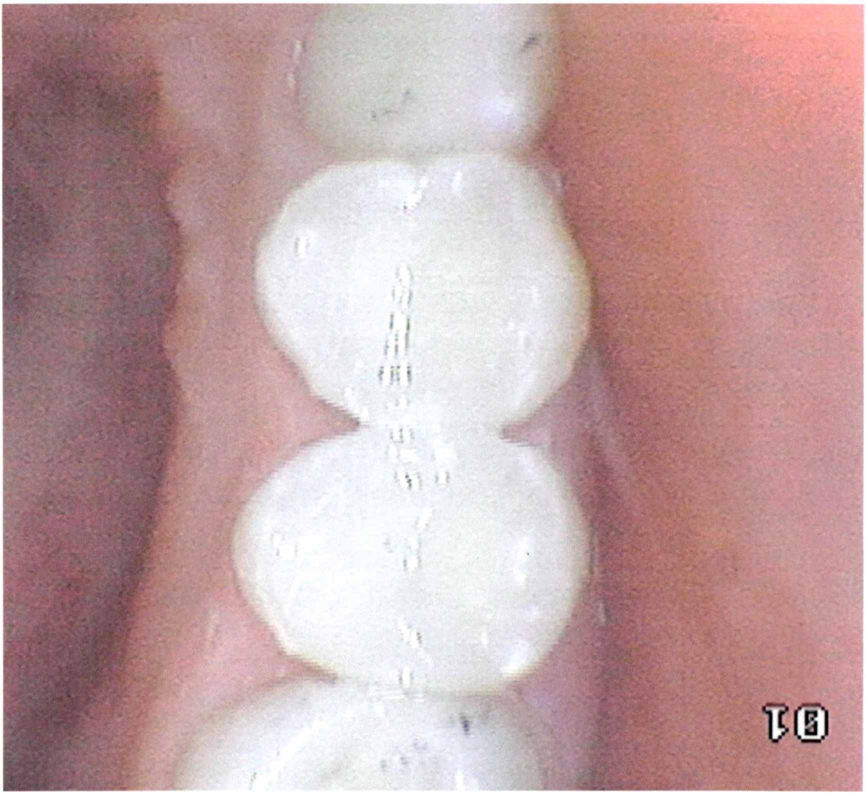

24DO, 25MOD and 26MO restored. Fillings with good contour and contact.

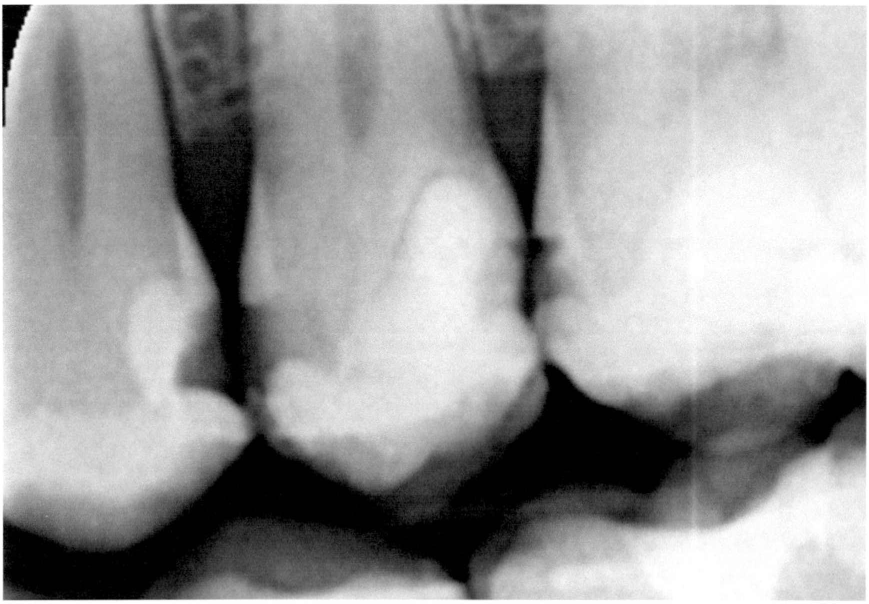

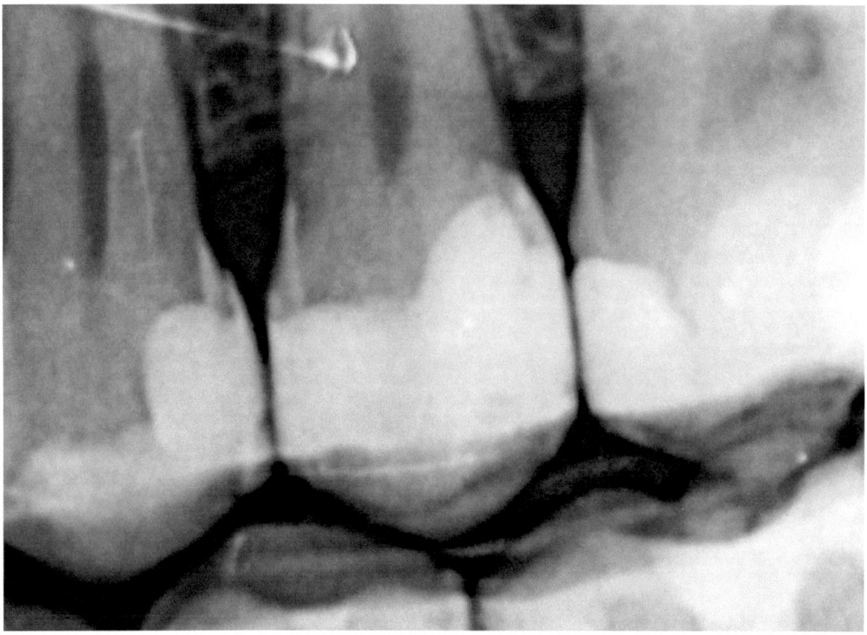

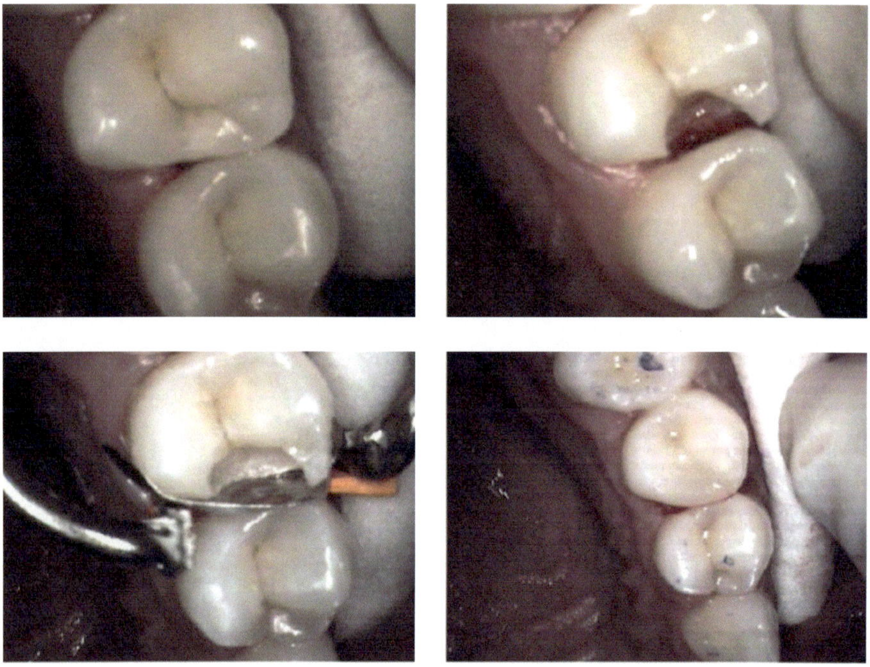

Again, use of Palodent sectional matrix, Bitine ring and inter-proximal wedge to obtain a good contour and a broad, tight contact.

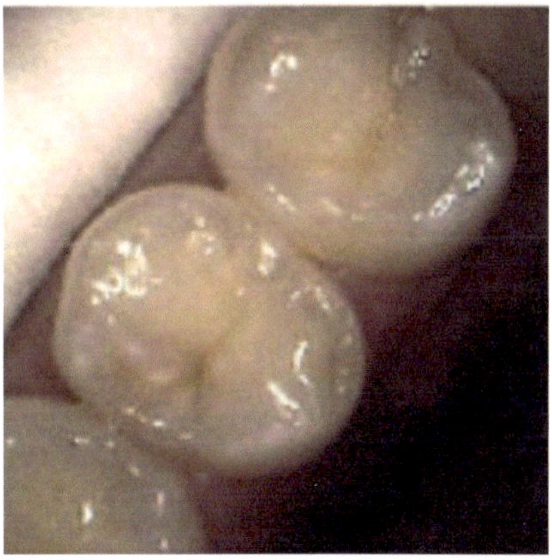
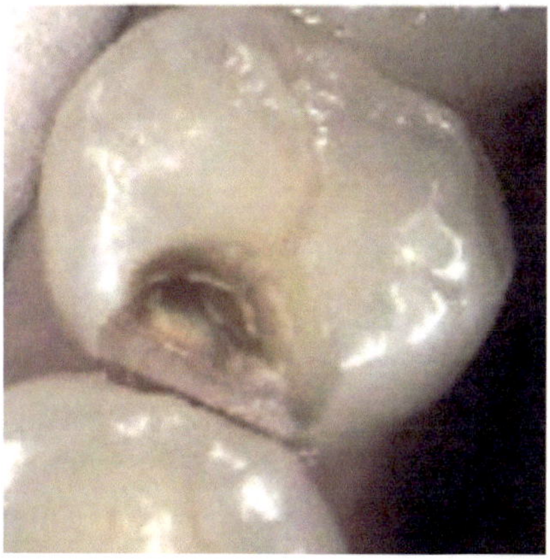
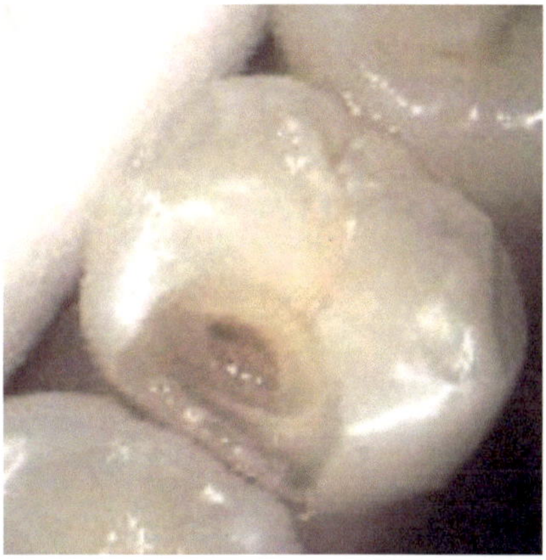
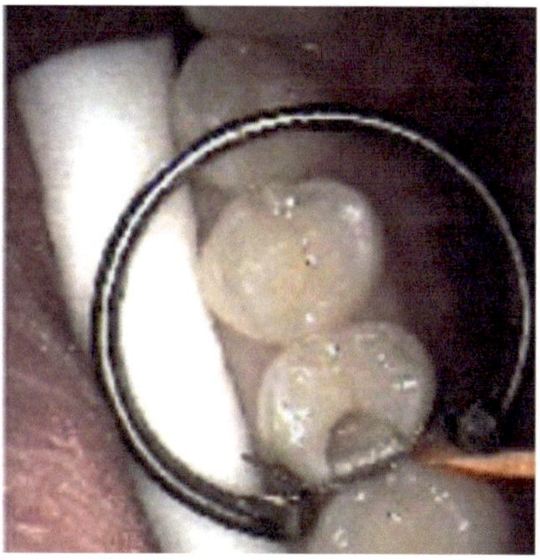
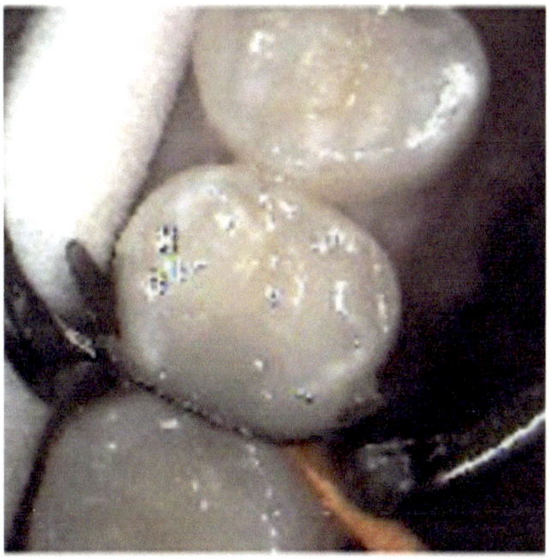
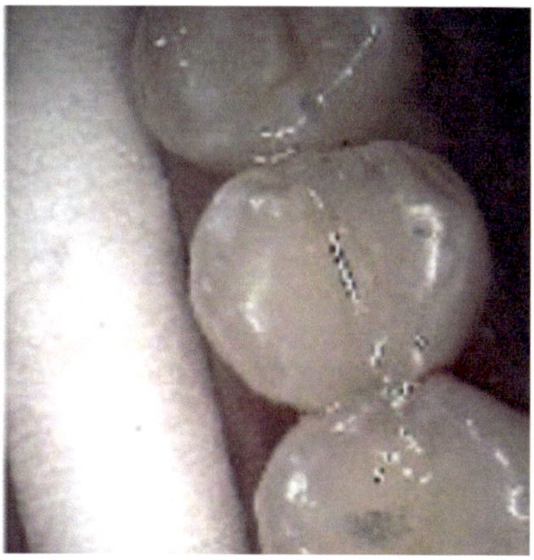

This page and the next twelve pages.

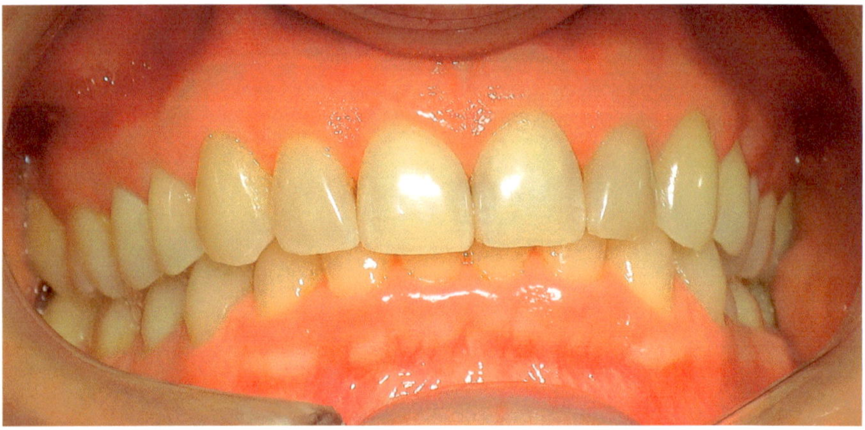

New patient, aged 33, brushing well, no symptoms.

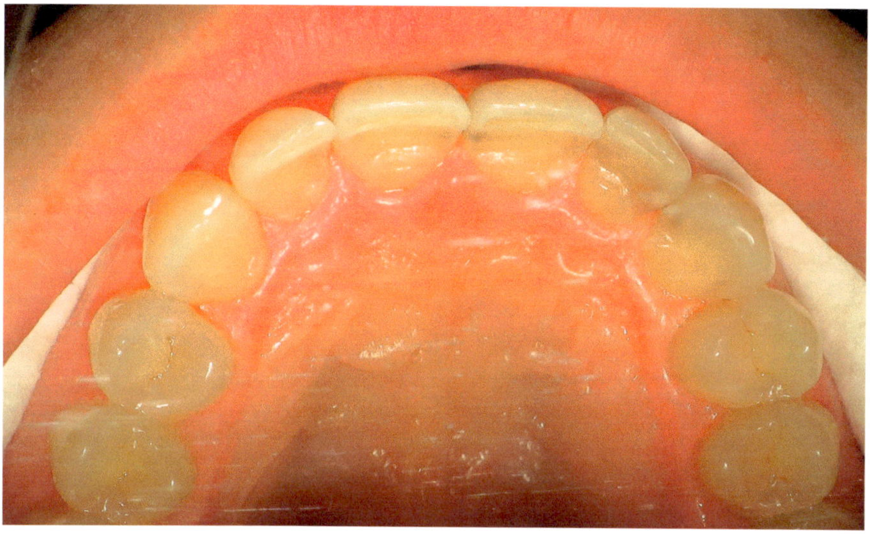

Clearly caries in a number of upper incisors and enamel lesions in many more.

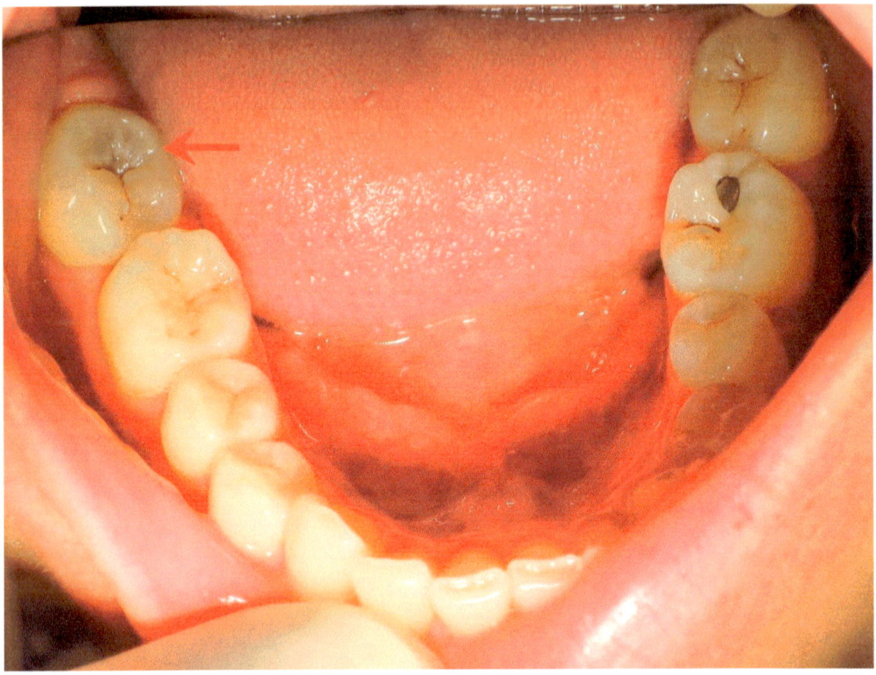

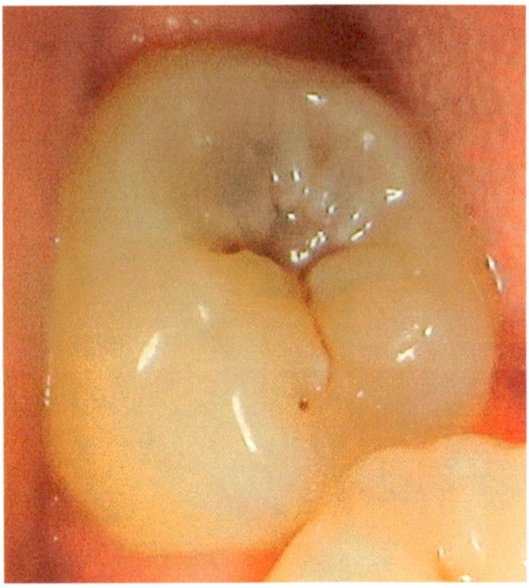

Same patient, slow spreading but deep caries in 47O. See the radiating dark discolouration beyond the fissure?

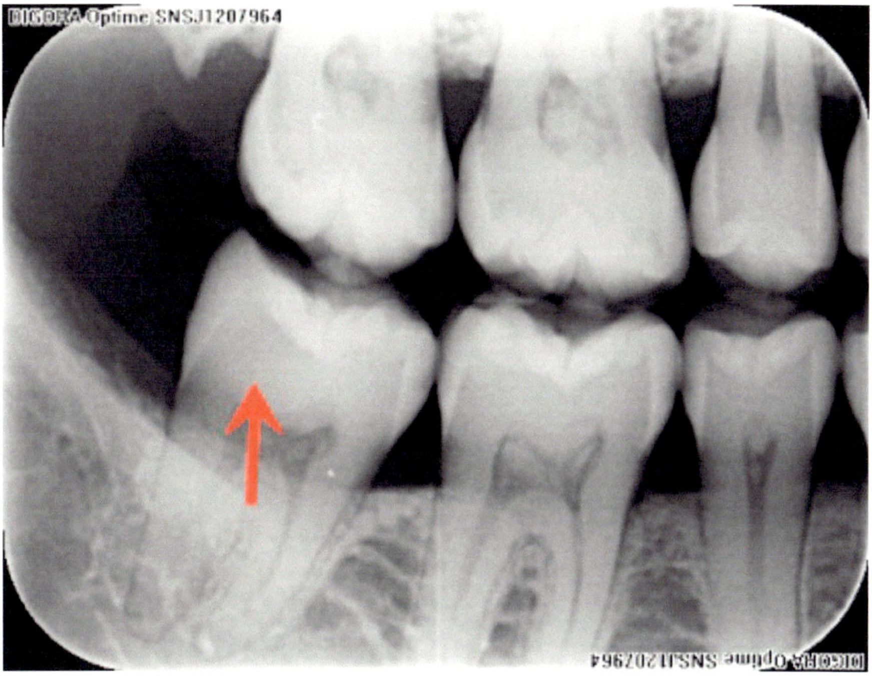


Same patient, the 47 occlusal caries that was seen clinically. Has lesions restricted within the enamel on 45D, 46M+D, 47M.

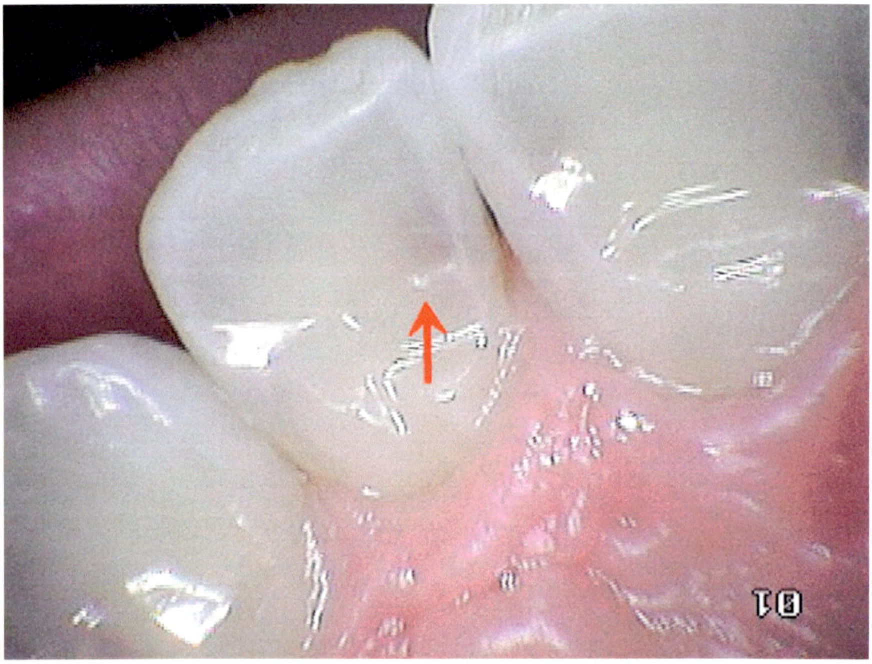


Caries 12M spreading along enamel-dentine junction and "mush-rooming" into the dentine.

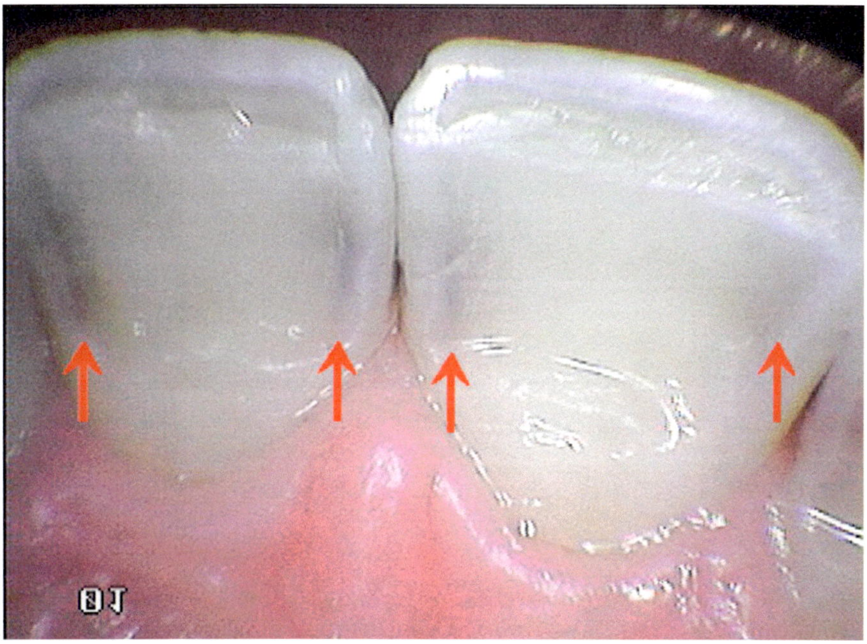

Caries spreading at enamel-dentine junction 11D, 11M, 21M and 21D.

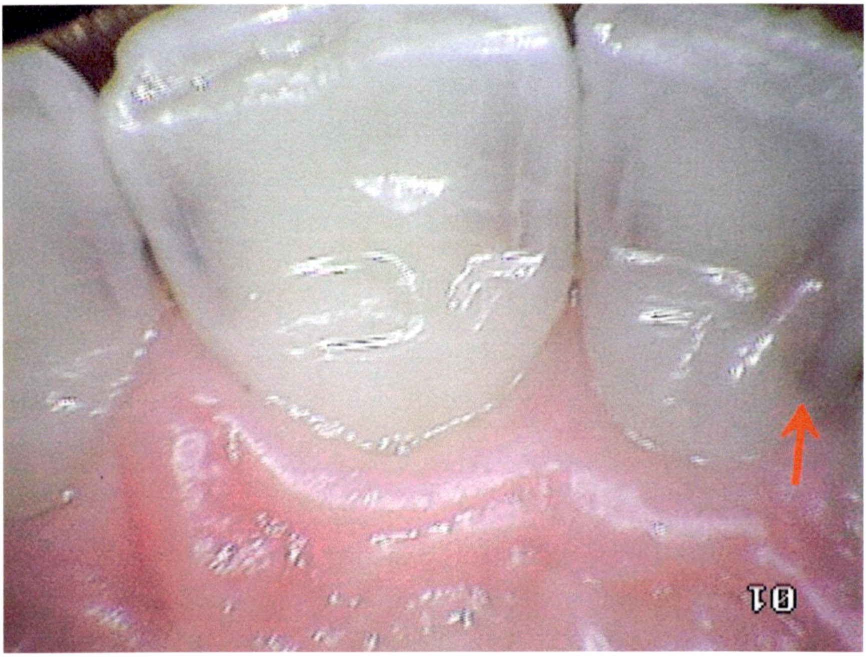

Interproximal caries. The decay in 22D is very deep.

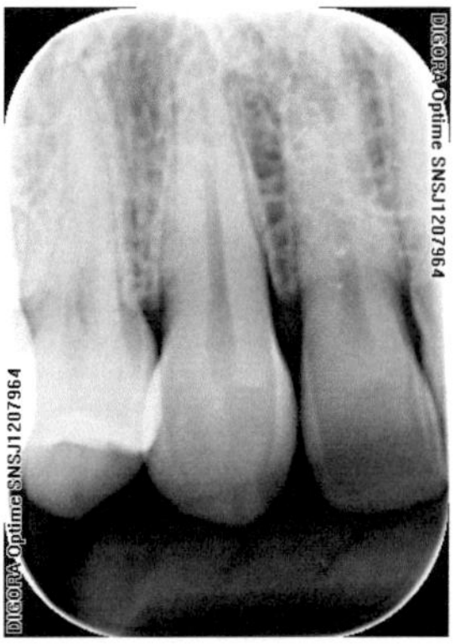


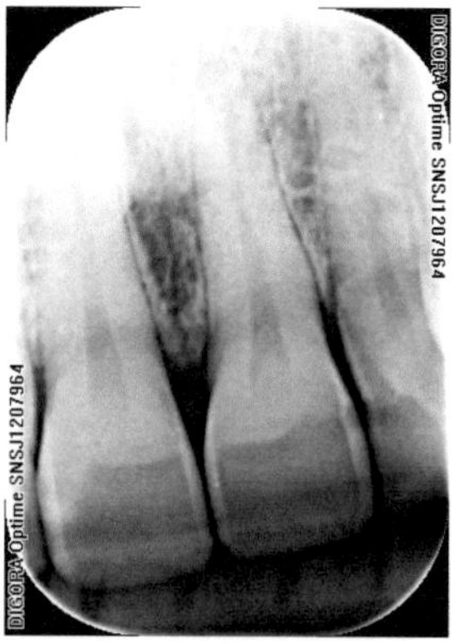


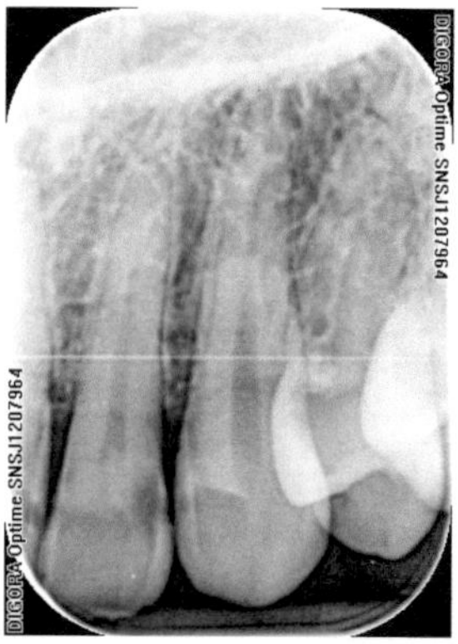


See how deep the caries in 22D is? Yet the patient has not had any symptoms. There has been no breakdown of tooth structure to the extent that the patient cannot feel any cavities.

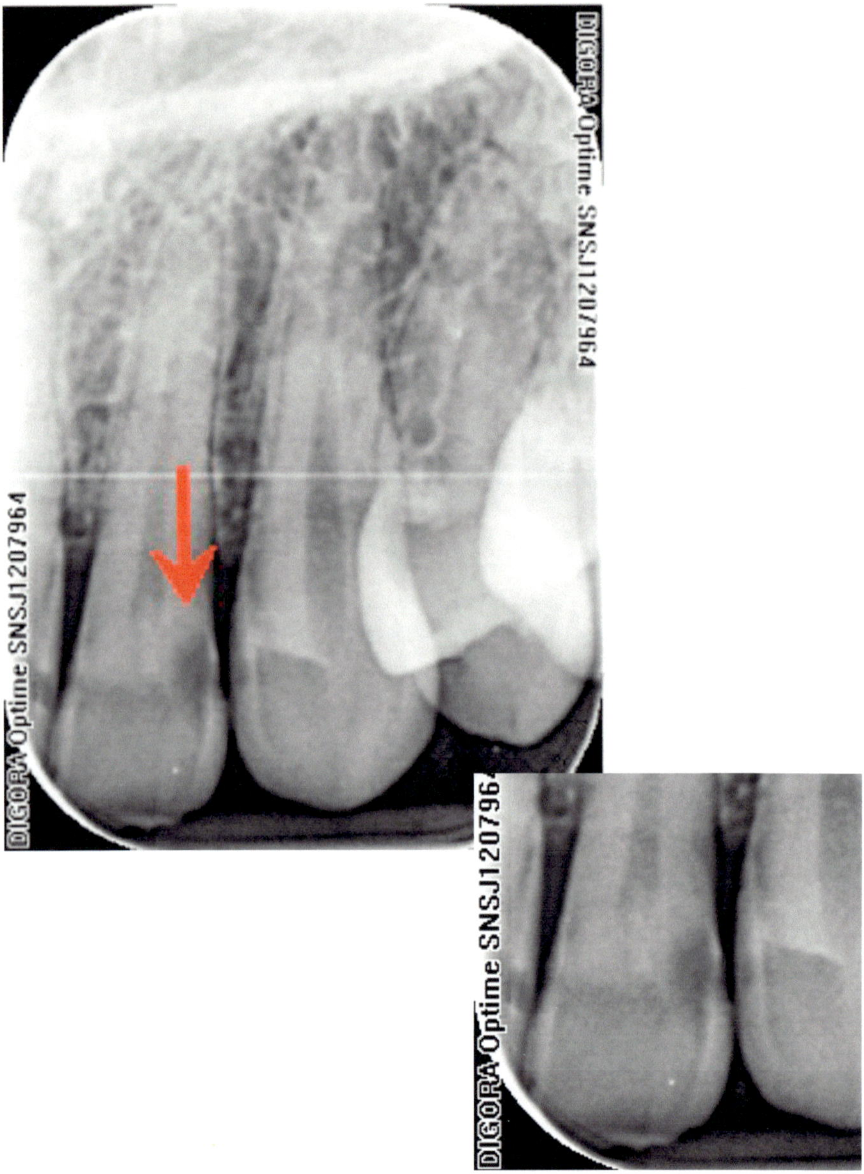


There is a possibility that the distal caries in 22 might involve the pulp. As such, caution the patient that the need for endodontic treatment may arise, even though there have not been any symptoms.

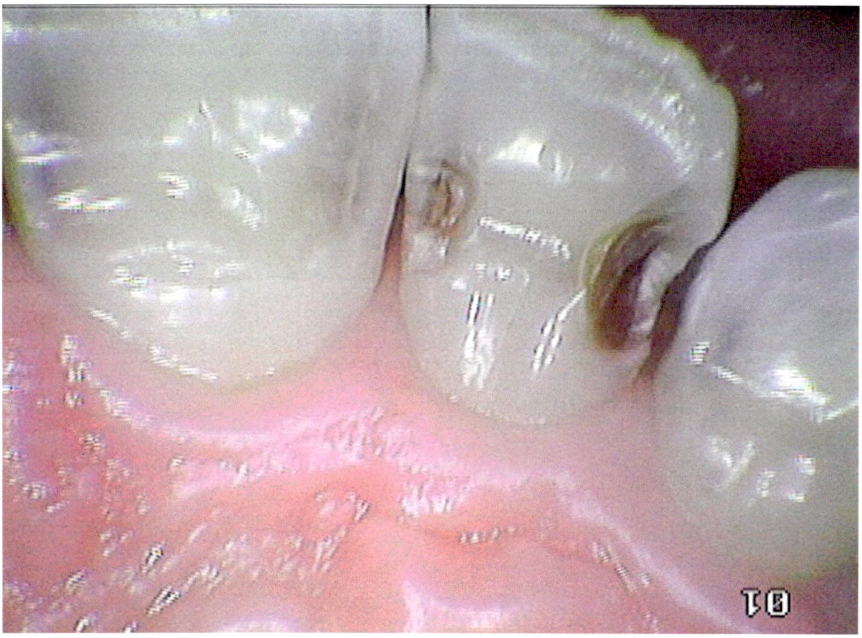

This picture was taken as we just went through the enamel, more for the patient's benefit as she could not feel holes and had no symptoms.

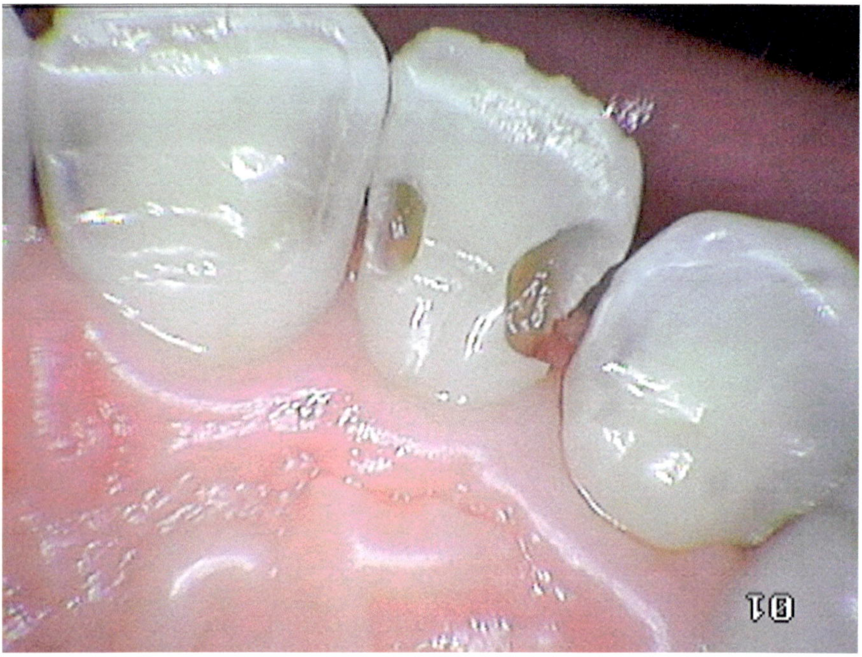


The cavities caries-free.

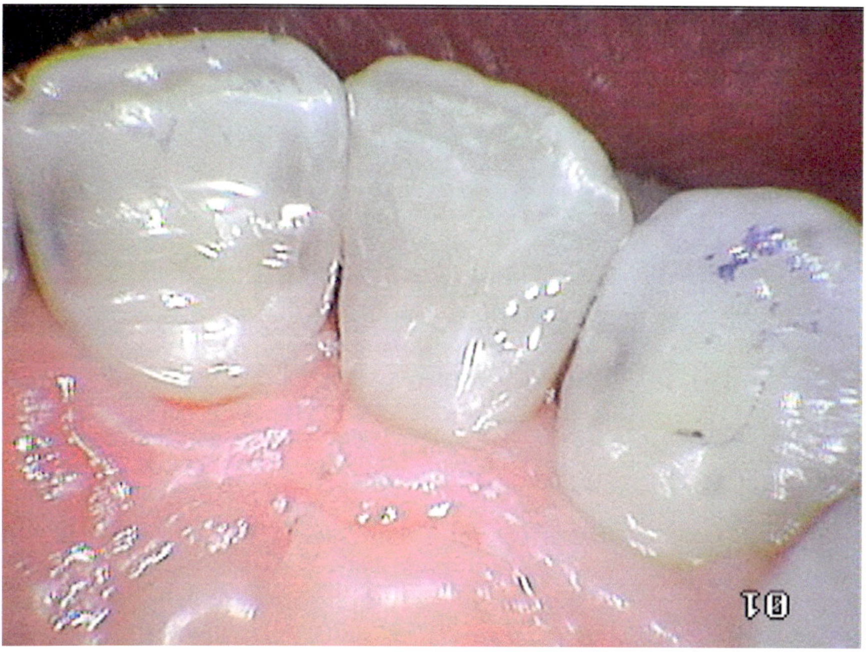

For that previous patient I knew exactly where there was dentinal involvement.

What I could watch.

Which teeth needed intervention.

And yet I took 9 photographs and 5 x-rays ..... WHY?

Because the patient could not feel even one cavity.

She had no symptoms of any sort.

She is seeing me for the first time.

She is in her mid-30s, may have seen other dentists regularly.

And here I am, a stranger, telling her she needs at least 5 fillings.

And possibly one root canal treatment.

That these cavities have been there for some time.

Can you imagine what is going through her mind?

The mistrust?

So the pictures are for her benefit, and to cover me.

Imagine if the 22, previously symptom-free, ached after I did the deep disto-palatal filling?

She'd come back and say "I was fine, what did YOU do to me?

....or "That filling YOU did...."

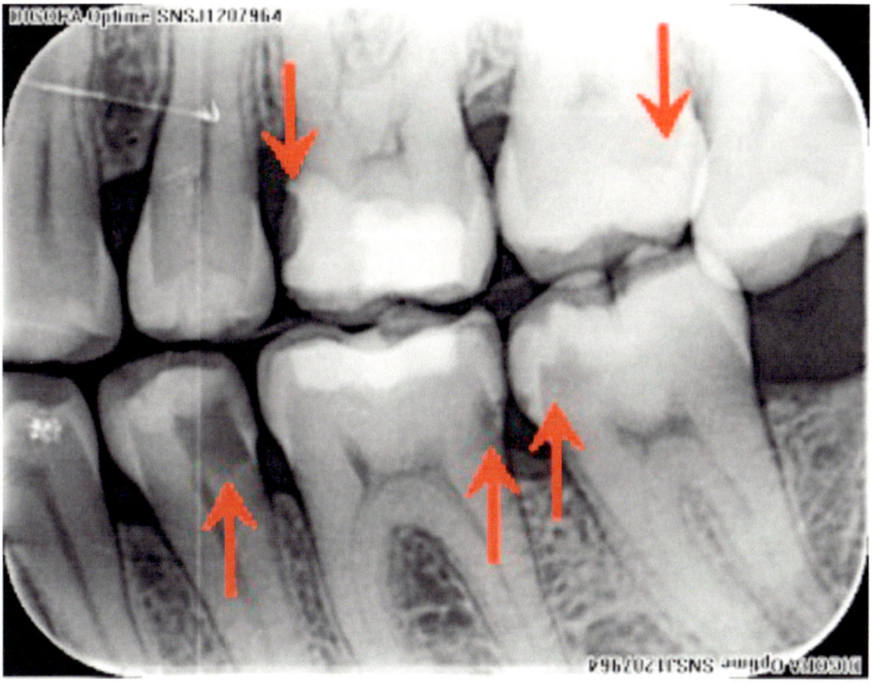

Lots to do. 26MOD, 27DO, extract 28, 37O, 36DO, 35 DO. 35 may require endodontic treatment.

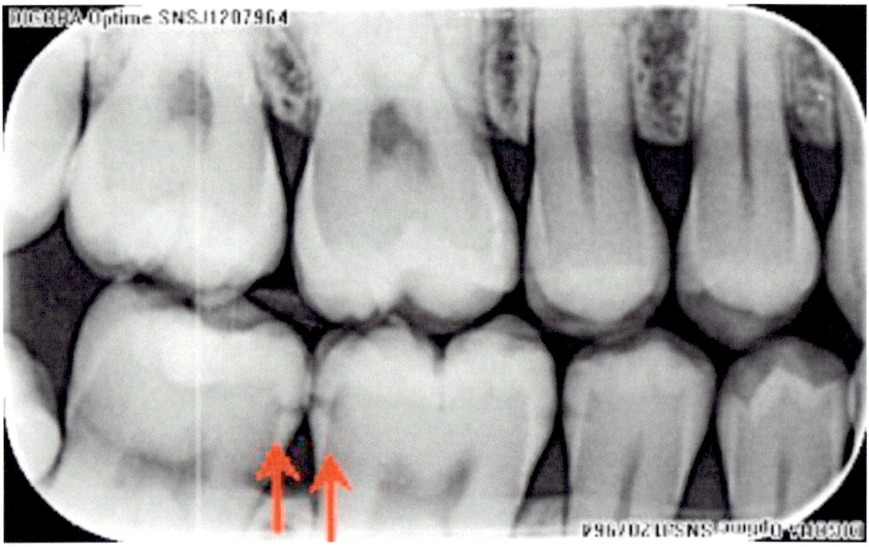

46DO and 47MO need filling. Monitor 46M, and 45D (possible early dentine involvement).

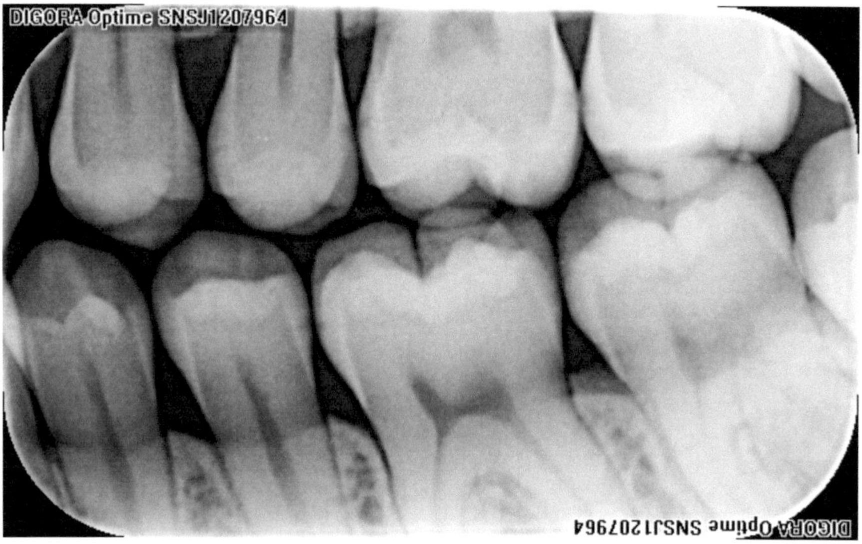


Can you spot 6 early enamel lesions?

Monitor 25D, 26M+D, 27M, 36M and 35D. 37 needs an occlusal filling.

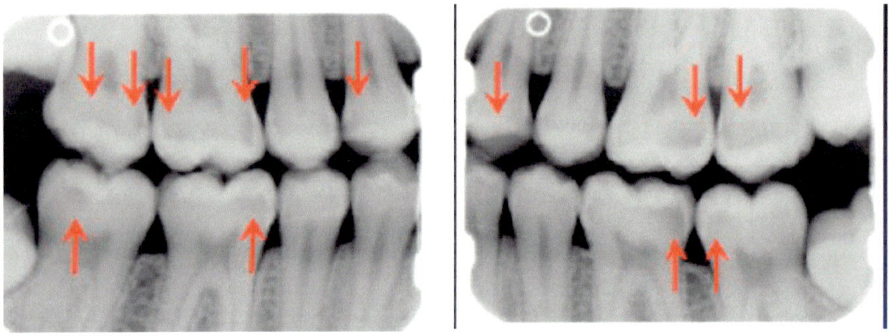

Before

Caries was attended to on 17O, 17MO, 16O, 16MO, 14DO, 25DO, 26O, 27MO, 37O, 36O, 46O and 47O.

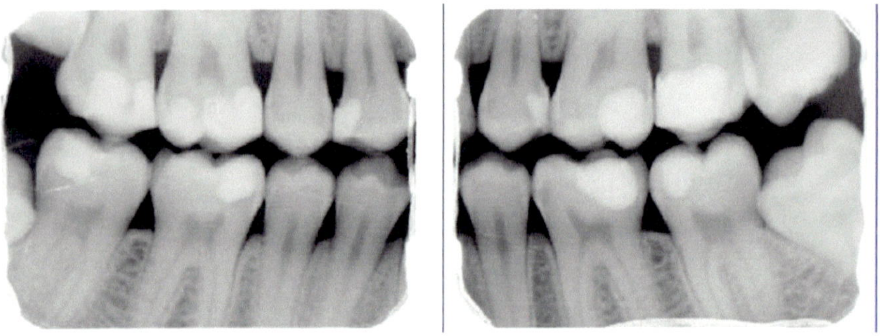

4 years later

All stable but 36M lesion has progressed, needs an MO. The depth of the fillings shows you that the caries is always larger than what the radiographs show you.

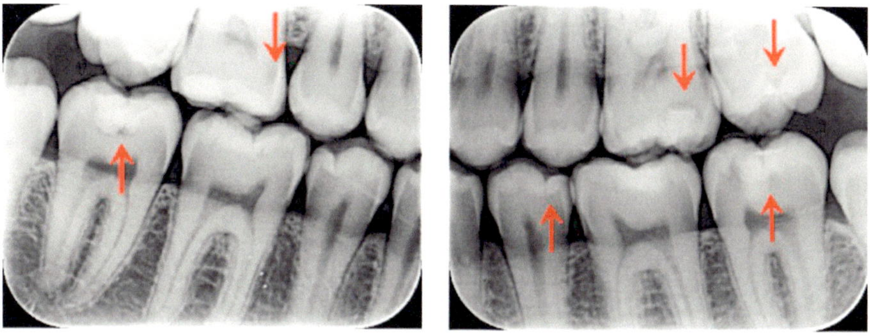

Before

Caries was found and then attended to on 16M, 26O, 27O, 37O, 35O and 47O.

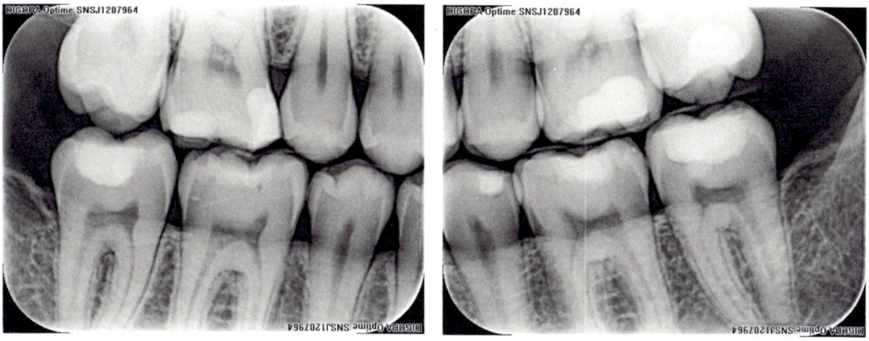


6 years later

The teeth are still good and stable, no new cavities and the alveolar crestal bone as healthy as before.

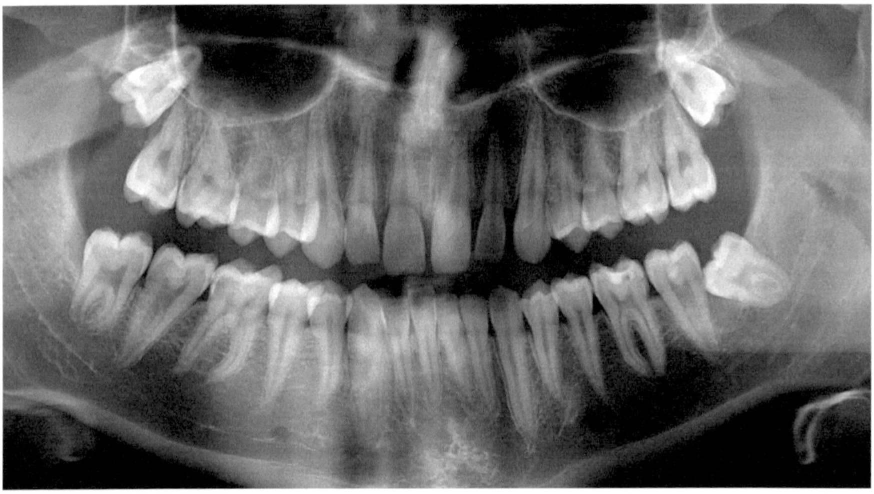

An OPG is great to have for your new patients to get an overview of the mouth, but you need intra-oral radiographs for more detail. See 46D here and in the bitewing to follow.

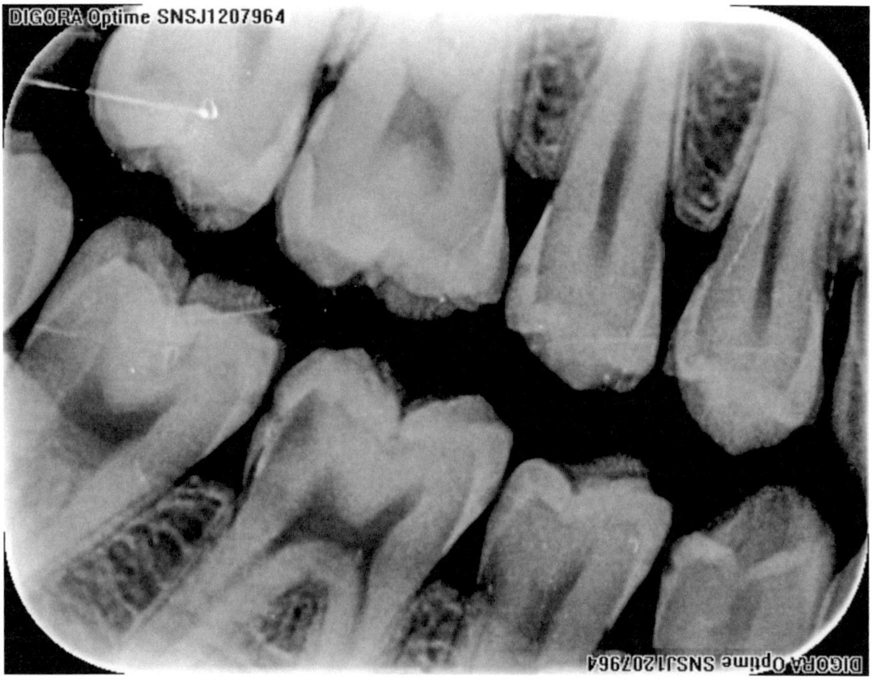


An OPG is great for a general overview, but you do need bitewing and periapical intra-oral radiographs for more detail.

Enamel lesions: 17M, 16D, 15D, 45D, and 46M.

Caries needing attention: 46O, 46DO, and 47O.

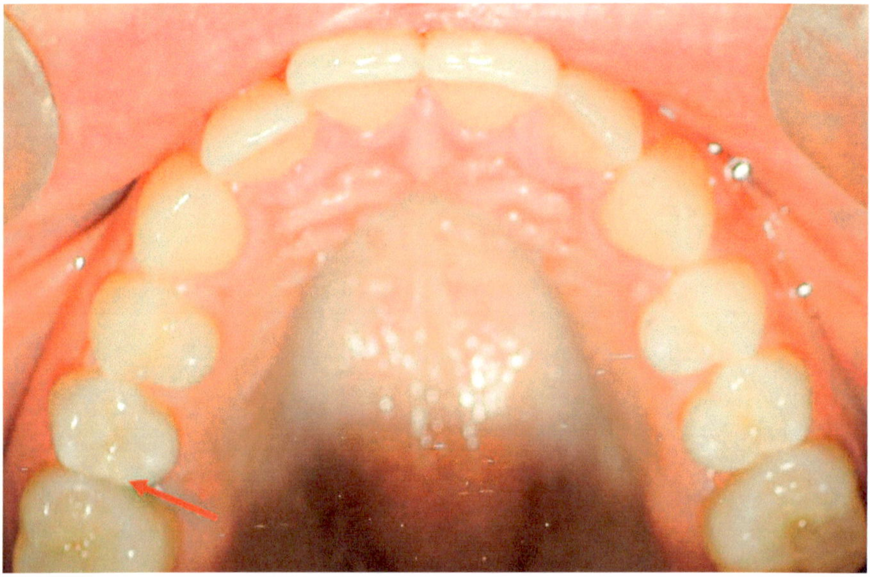

15 distal caries

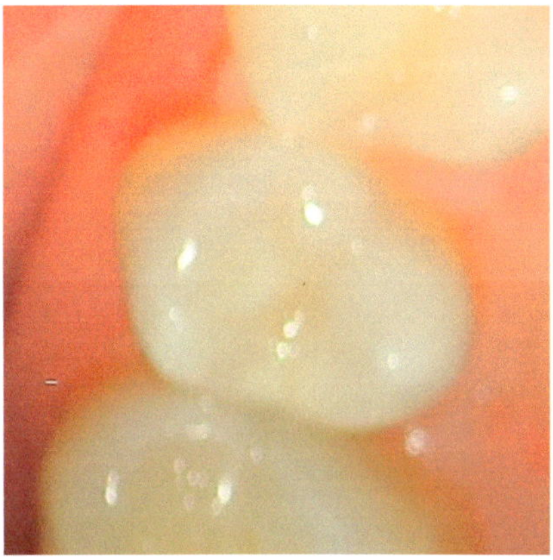

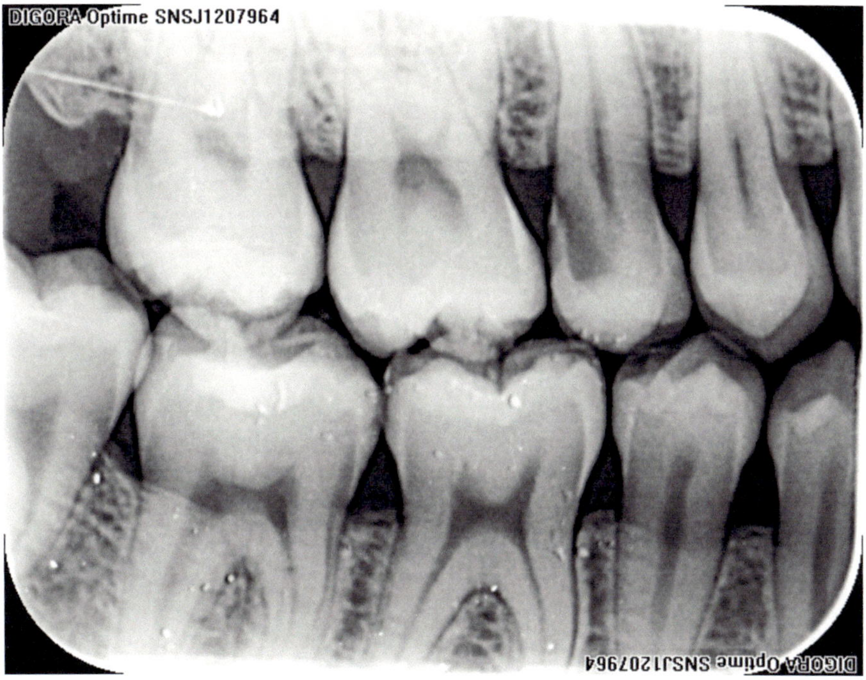


Had you not seen the cavity in 15D clinically, and not taken a right bitewing radiograph, you would miss this very deep cavity. What might at this stage be just a filling would become a need for endodontic treatment as well.

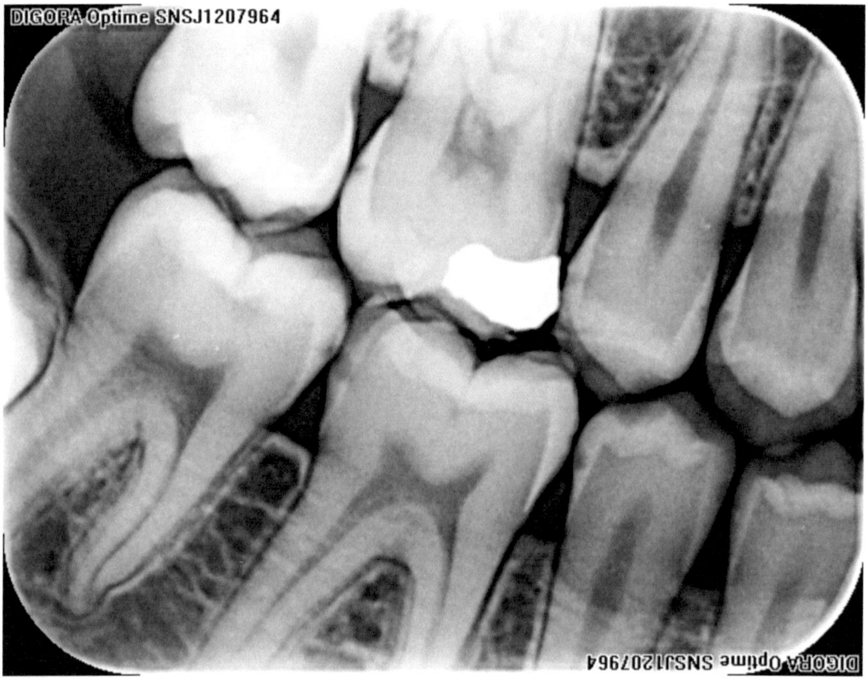


To do: 17O, 46DO, 47O.

To monitor: 16D, 15D+M, 14D, 45D, 46O and 47M.

Borderline: 15D – how does it look clinically?

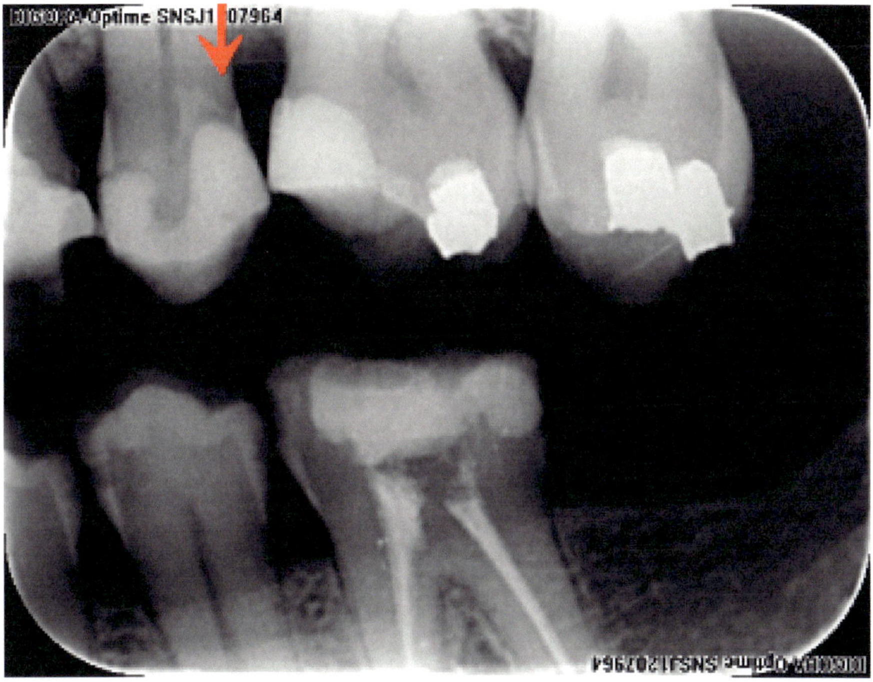


Apart from the clear problems in 35M, and for 36 to be assessed for a crown, have a careful study of 25, which appears to have caries beneath the resin filling. How does the tooth look clinically?

Perhaps the tooth had a MOD amalgam which was removed, the cavity cleaned and the tooth filled. The secondary dentine shows there has been long term chronic irritation, which could be from the past rather than the present. If there are no symptoms and no clinical indication, is this a tooth one would monitor, with a follow up radiograph 18 months to 2 years later? Or do you replace the MOD filling now?

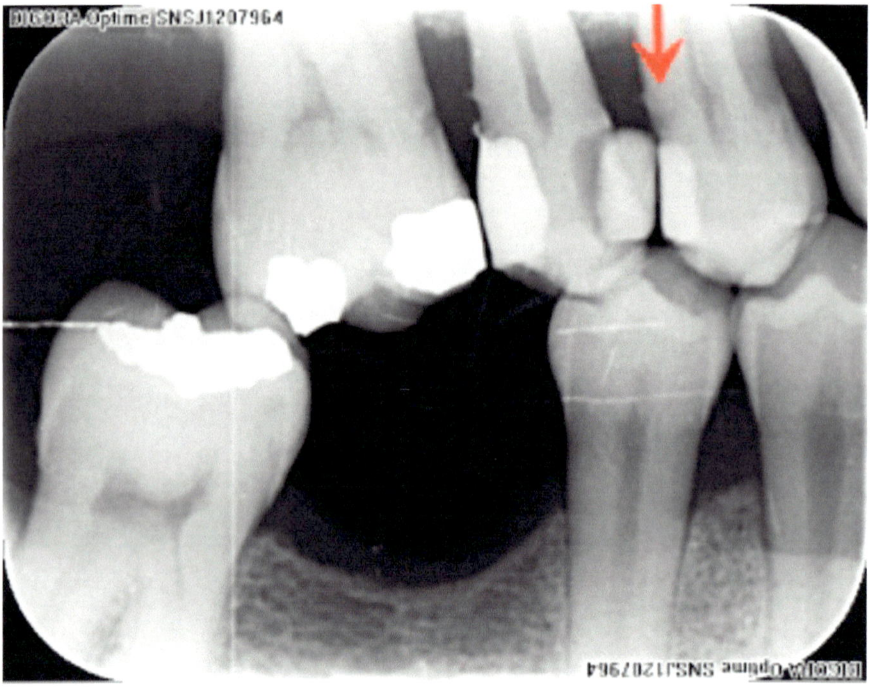


You would certainly want to probe 14 distal-cervical when fixing 15.

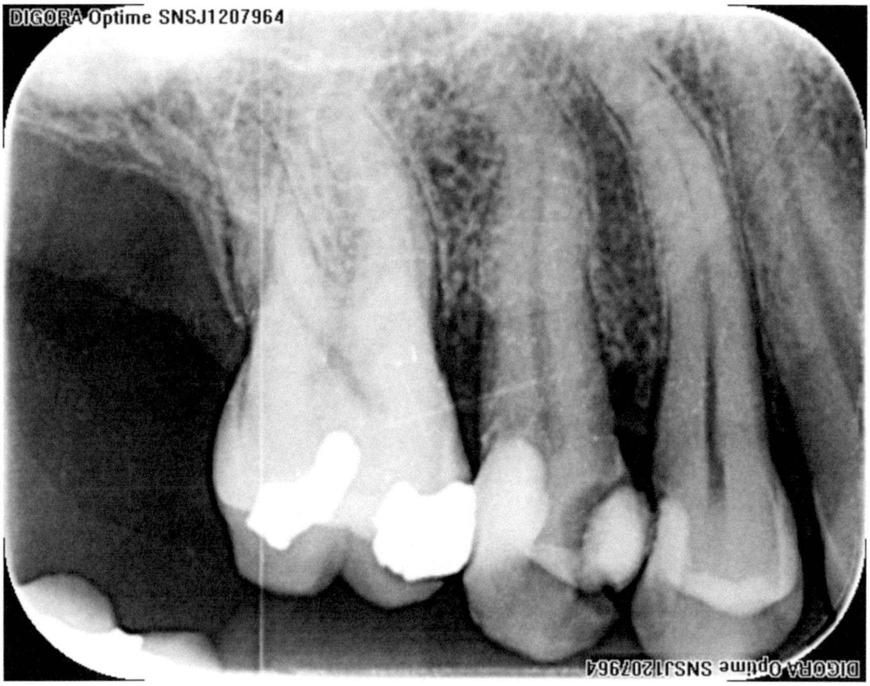


No periapical pathology is seen on 14 and 15.

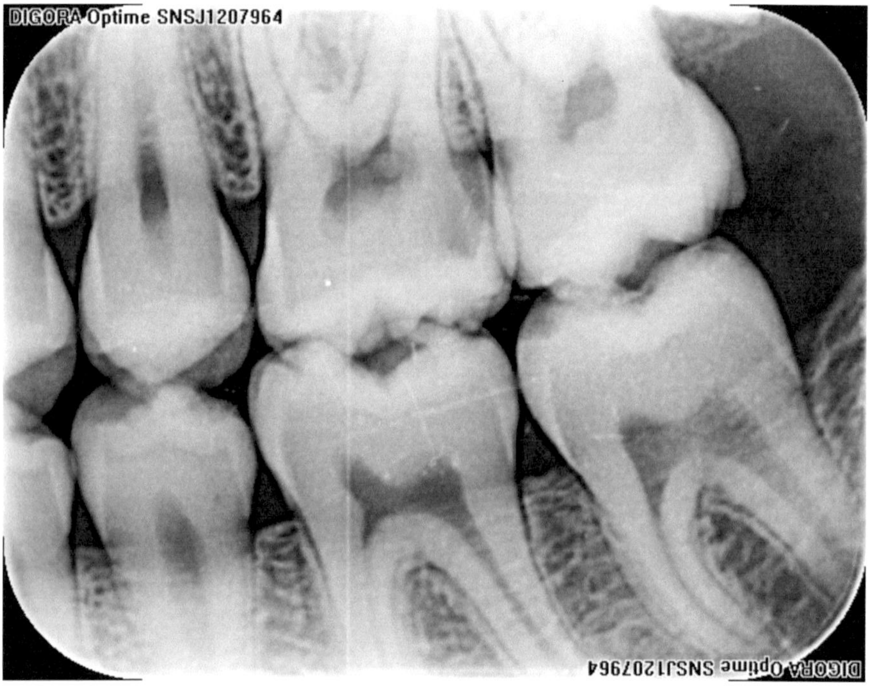


26 has very deep distal caries.

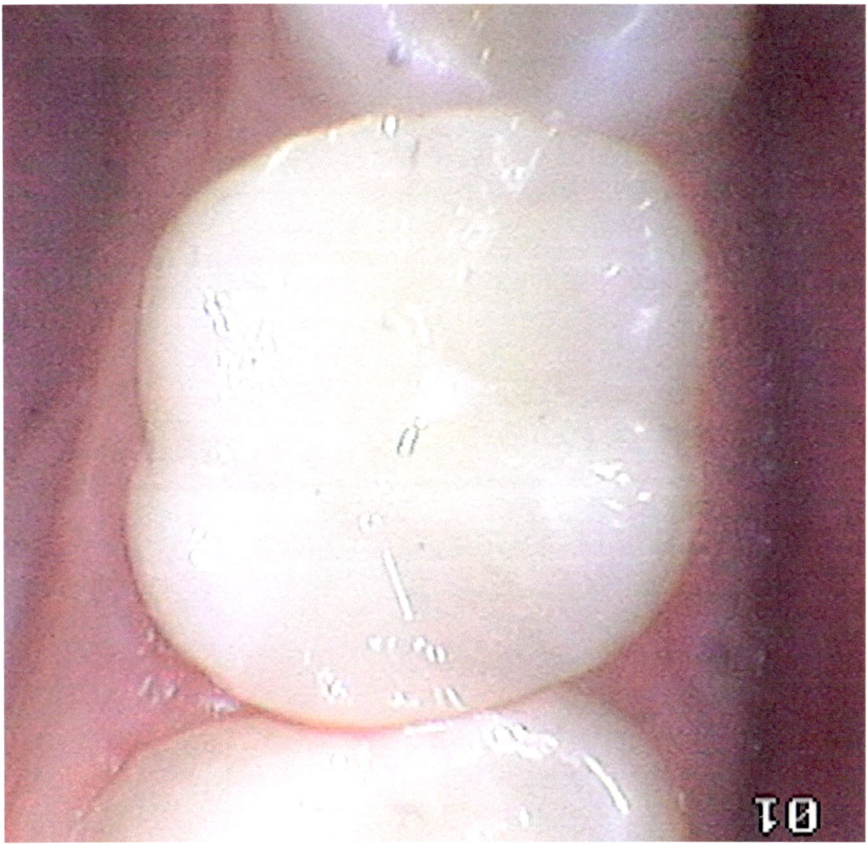

The 26DO cavity restored.

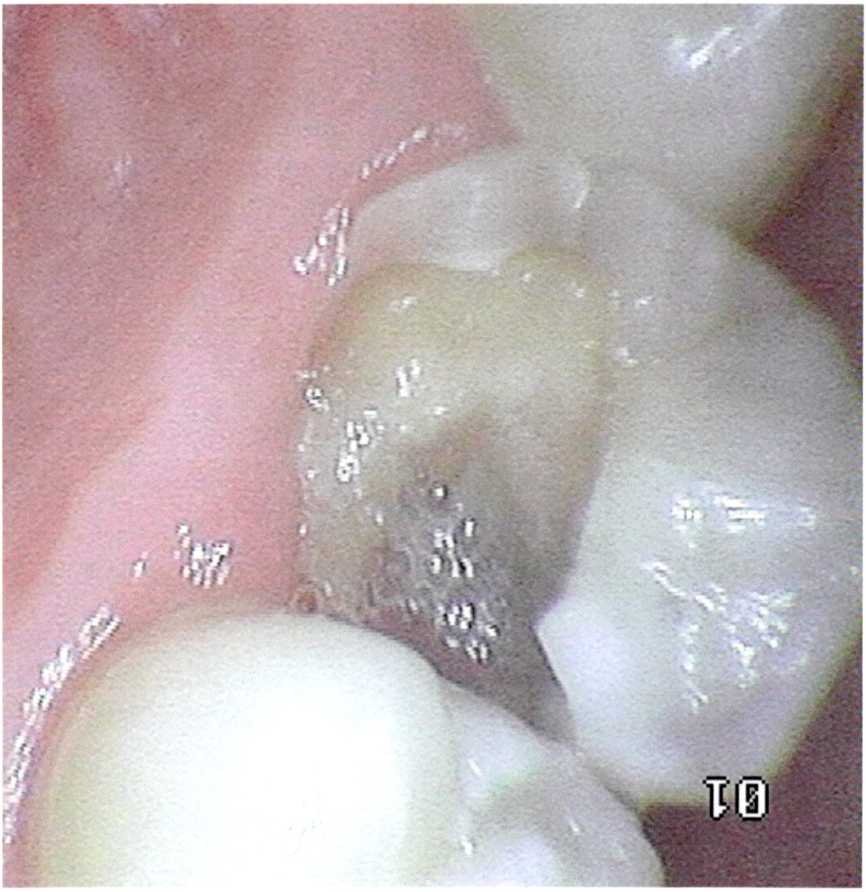


If this patient does not want to lose this tooth, send him/her away. You are not a miracle worker. Anything you do other than an extraction will come back to haunt you.

It has rapidly spreading caries, there is extensive loss of tooth structure, it is carious to subgingivally and possibly even to the alveolar crestal bone level.

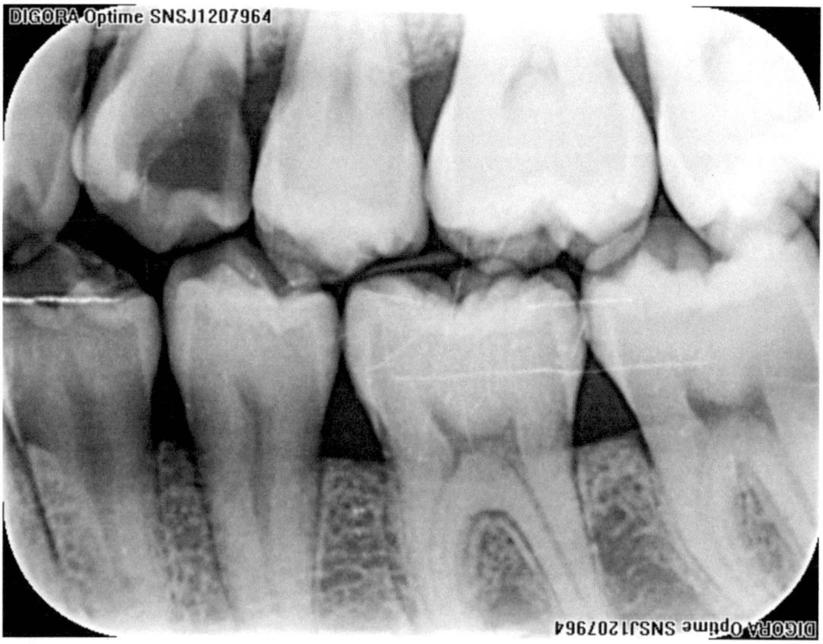


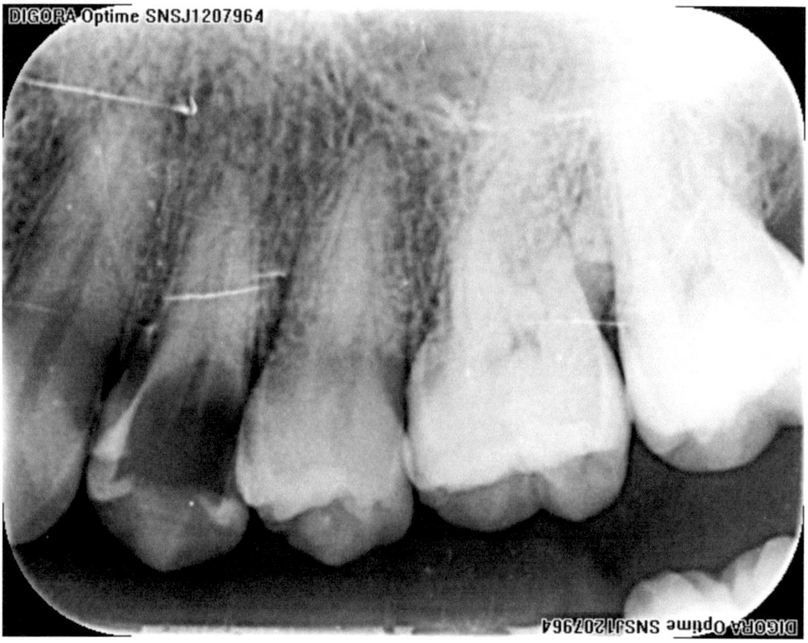


There is only one choice for 24 – extraction.

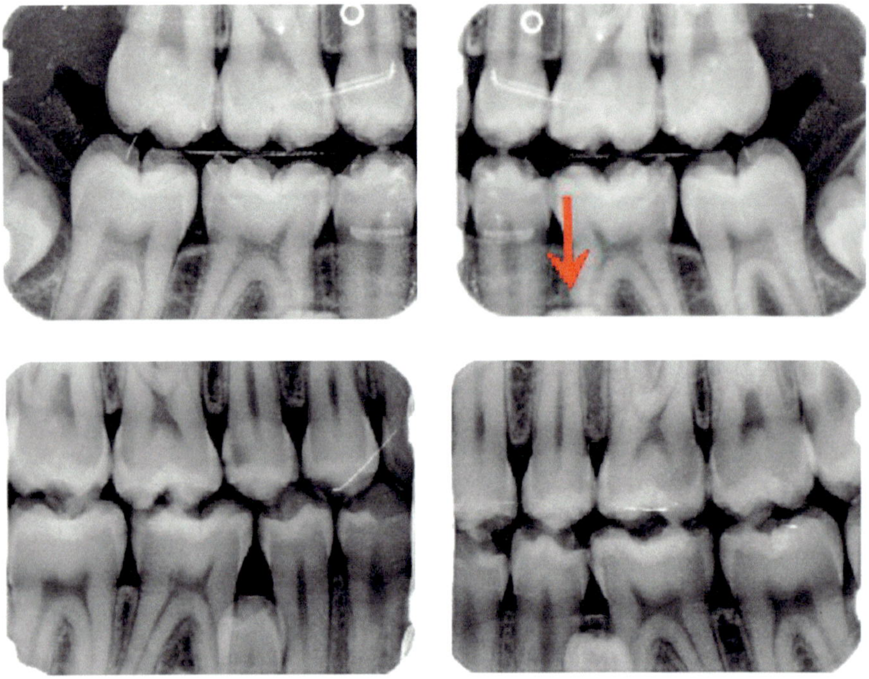

When you take bitewings, look at everything, not just for caries. The old left bitewing (top picture) hinted at something low down between 35 and 36. Later bitewings (lower pictures) show super-numerary teeth between 35-36 and 45-46. Note also that 16D and 15D have developed interproximal caries.

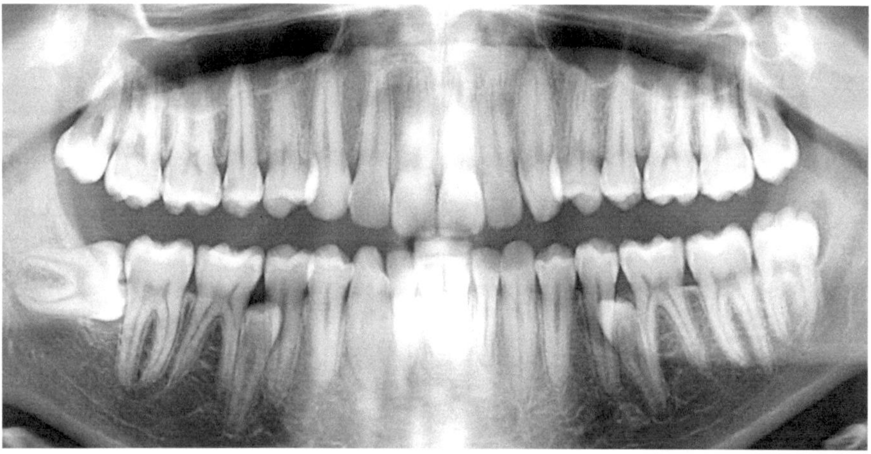

Having seen supernumerary teeth on the second (later) set of bitewings, it is important to investigate further by having an OPG done. This shows supernumerary teeth between 35-36 and 45-46, almost like a second set of second premolar teeth.

Before

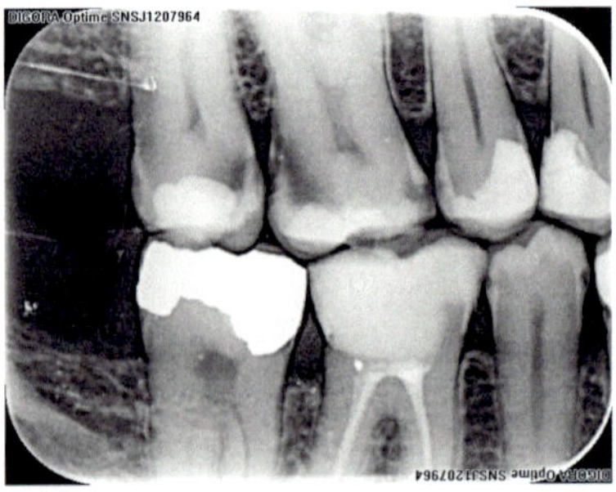


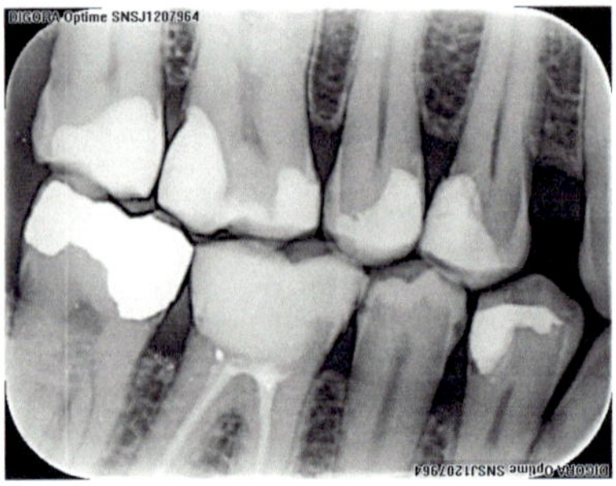


After

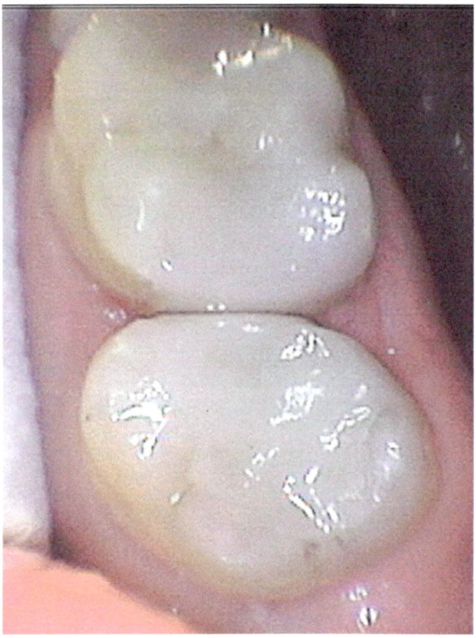

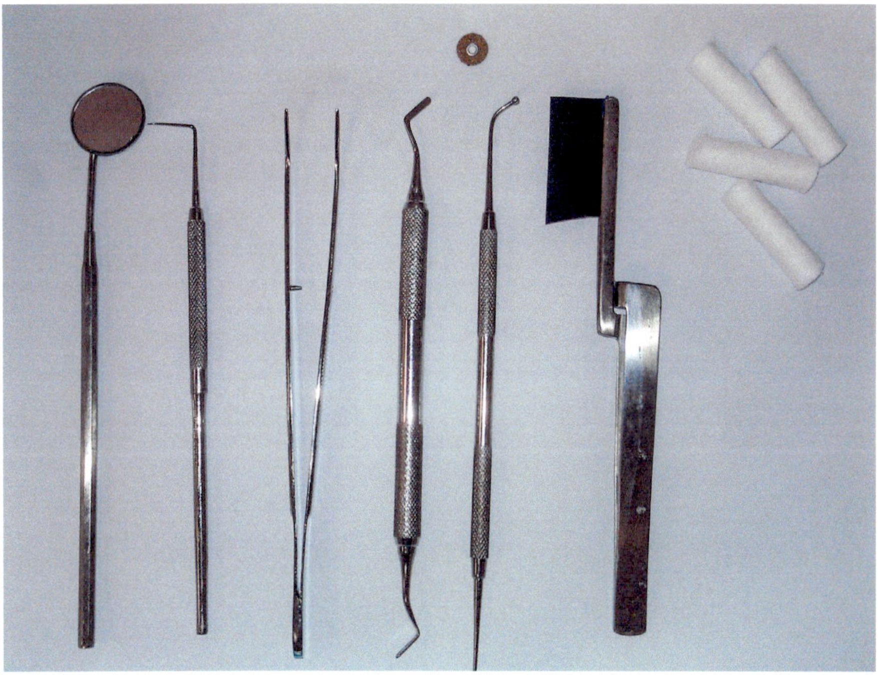

Example of a standard instrument tray for restorative work.

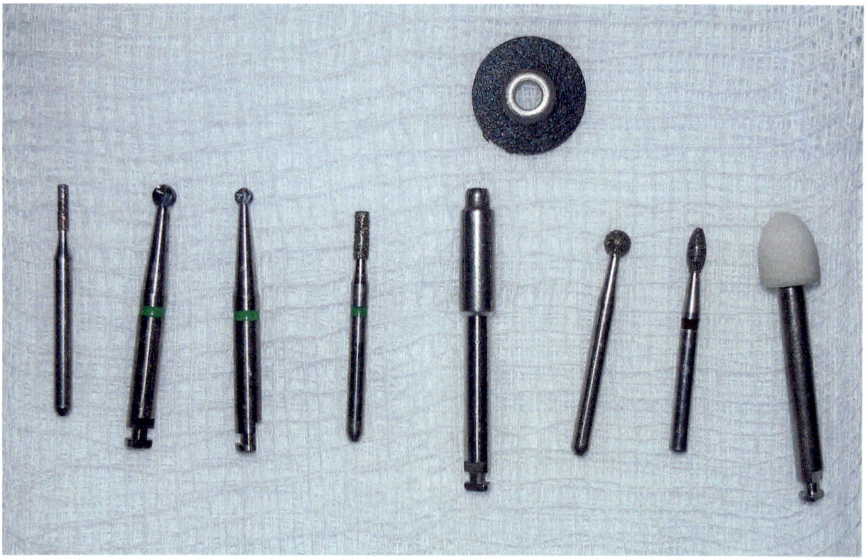

Example of bur set used for all the restorative work you see in this book.

This page and the next two pages.

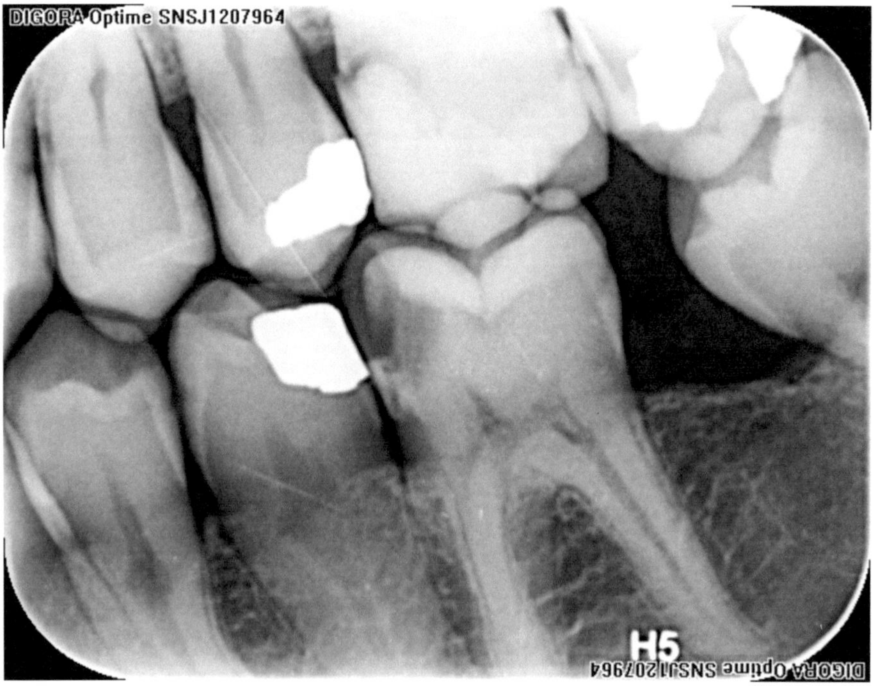


This emergency patient presented for attention to 36.

## Copy of My Clinical Notes:

c/o lost filling lower left 2 weeks ago, no pain.

Had a temporary filling placed 3 years ago and never went back.

Has no symptoms to hot or cold, no aching.

Limited o/e shows 36 has a deep MOB cavity.

No TTP, no tenderness b → l pressure, no tenderness buccal sulcus.

L BW shows cavity 36MOB is deep - showed pt and told him most likely will need just a filling but caries is close to pulp. Will know more when the cavity is clean.

Will work on 36 today.

Recommend return for a comprehensive oral exam.

For OPG.

2ml 3% Scandonest Plain LA.

36 Theracal, Prelude, Dyract Extra A2, very deep mesially and deeper still occlusally (Theracal placed here).

Cautioned pt if achy initially not to be concerned as cavity was deep.

Told of the possibility that the tooth may require root canal treatment in future.

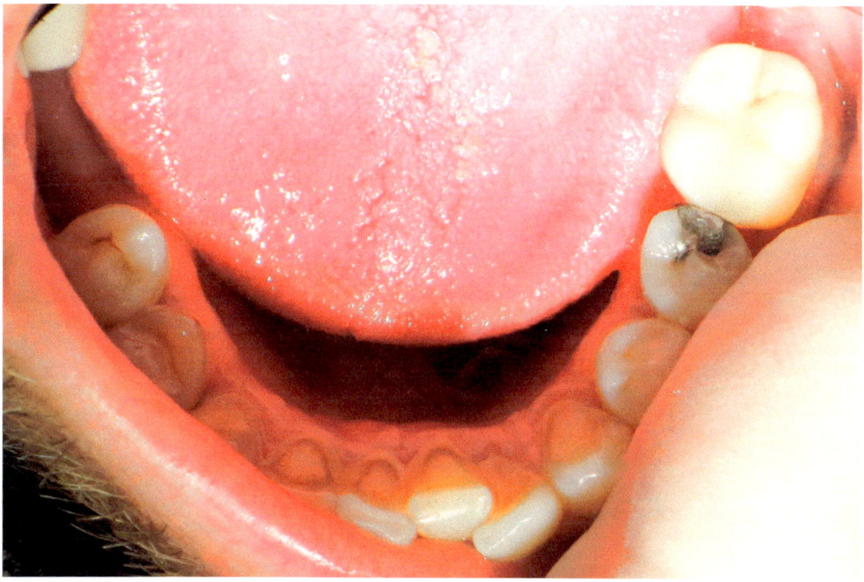

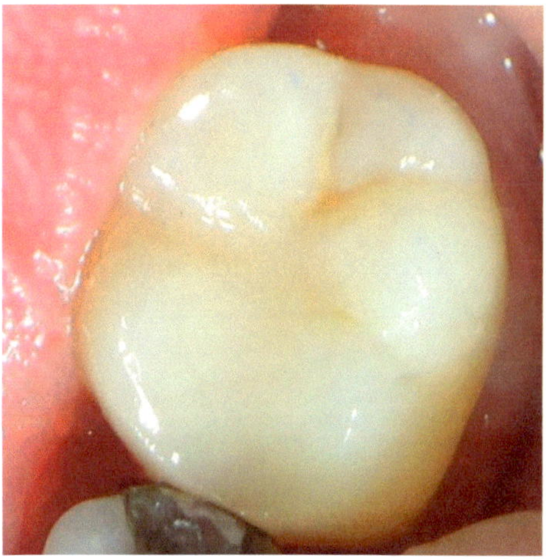

Fill out medical history form, talk to patient, limited oral examination, discuss, left bitewing x-ray, discuss, consensus, treat.

The tooth 36 restored.

# THE POWER OF *Floss*

December 2016

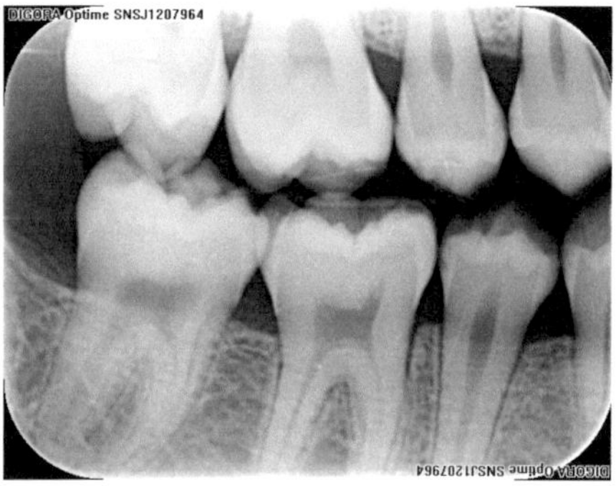


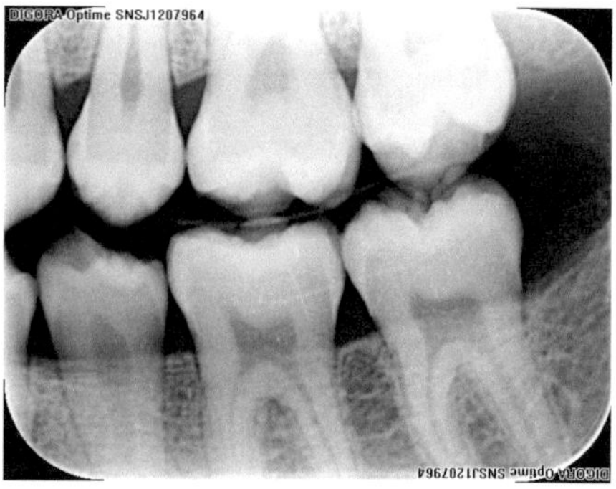


November 2018

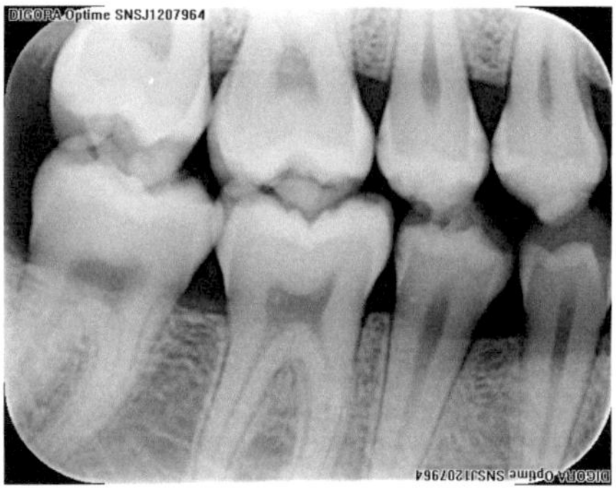


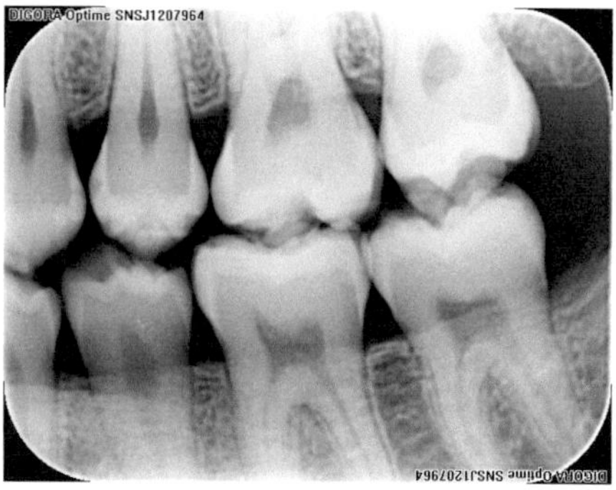


Son – uses dental floss

December 2016

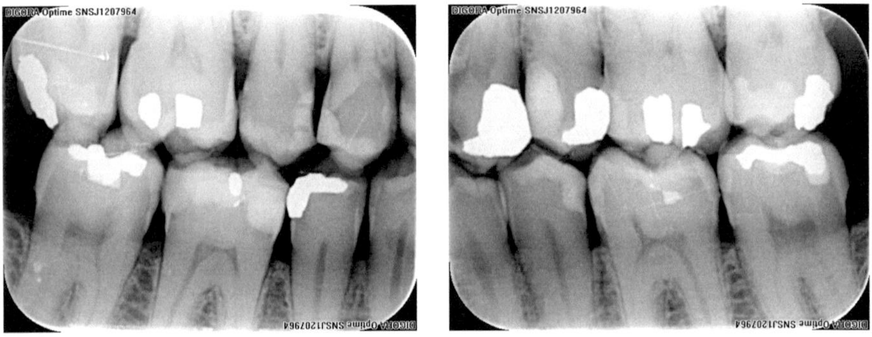


November 2018

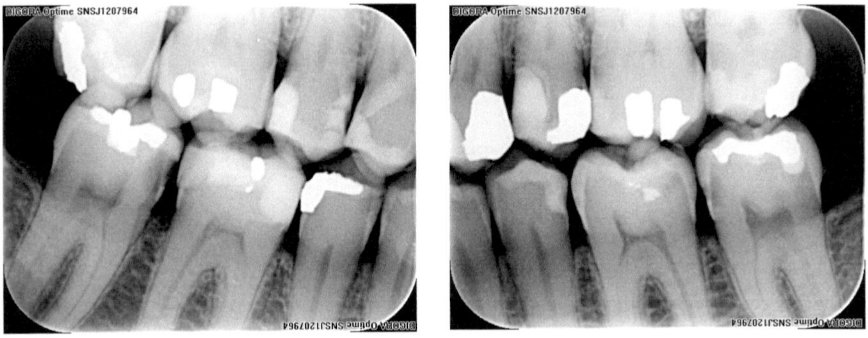


Father – does not floss
Has 9 interproximal fillings, and needs two more,
on 37M and 47M

*Tell all your patients to ...*

# "ONLY FLOSS THE TEETH YOU WANT TO KEEP!"

*Recurrent*
CARIES

*Secondary*
CARIES

*Impacted*
TEETH

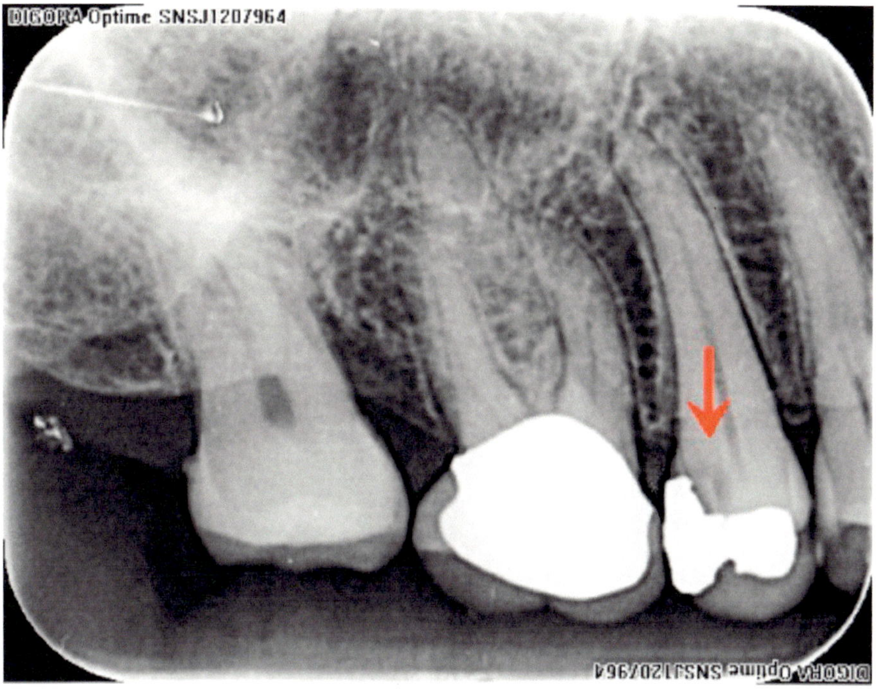


Cracked fillings can be a result of deep caries beneath – see 15DO amalgam filling.

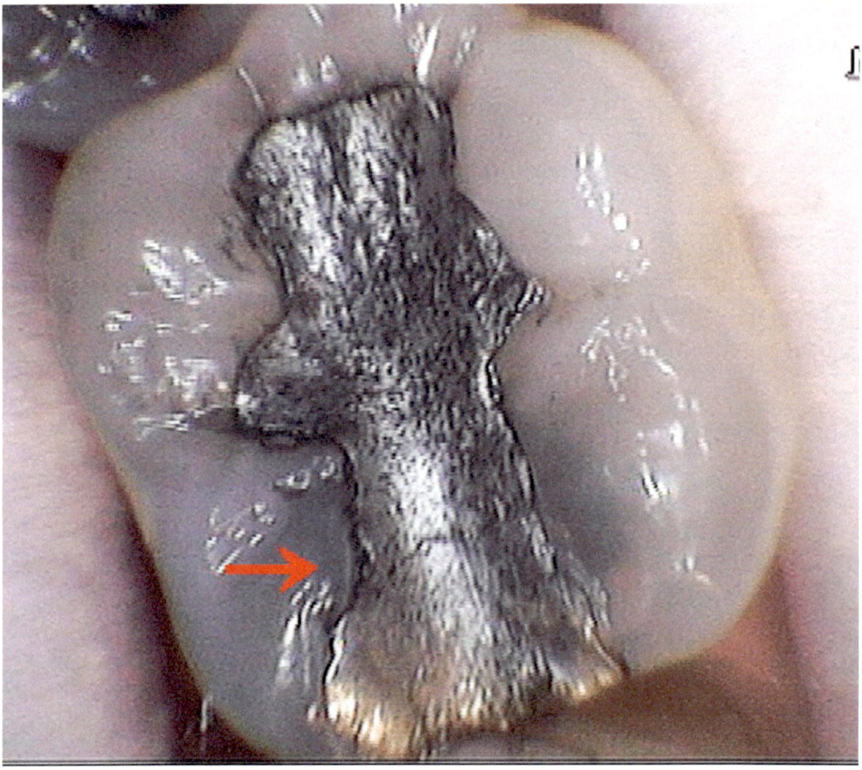

Crack in 46MO amalgam filling.

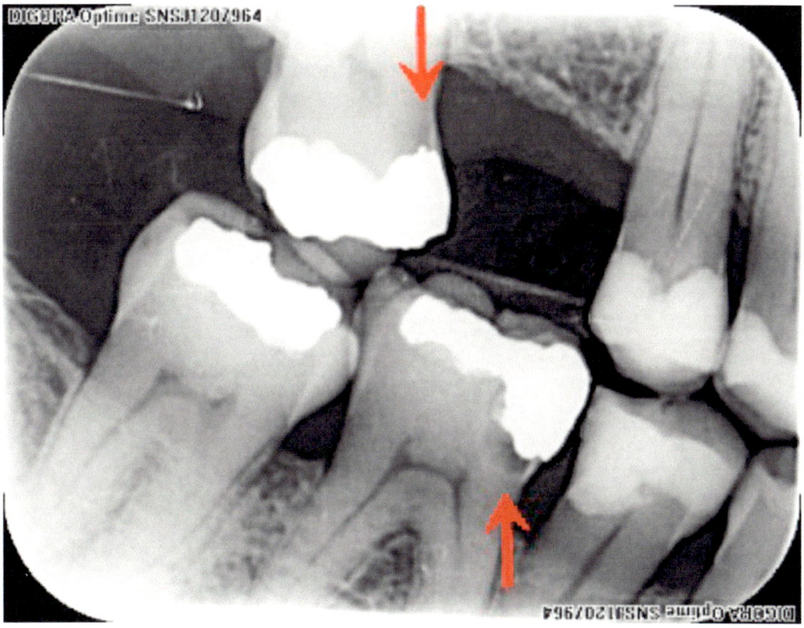


46 has deep secondary caries beneath the fractured MO amalgam filling. See also the deep caries mesially beneath the 17MO filling.

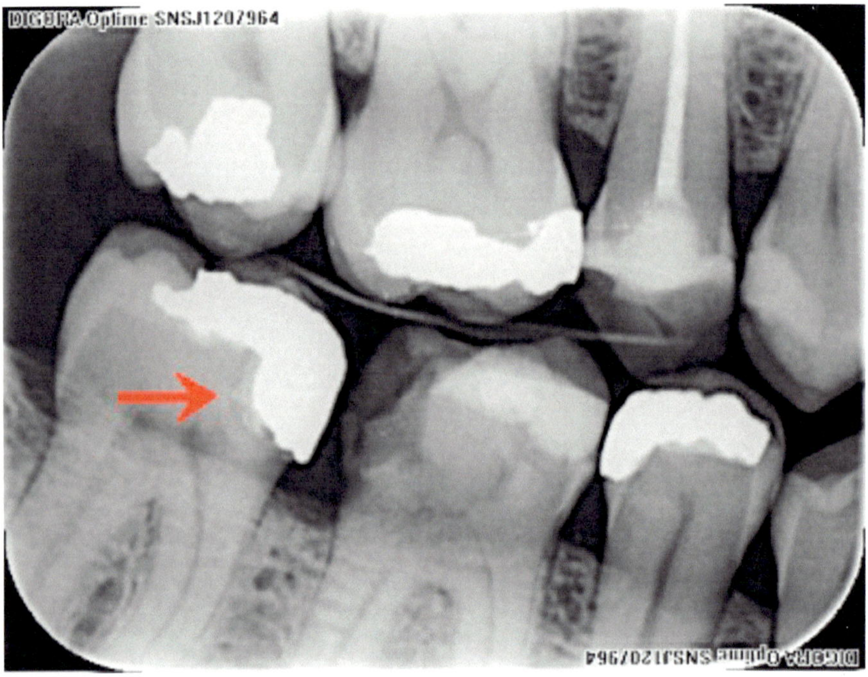


Patient presented with a broken filling on 46. The appearance of 47 indicates that if you remove the filling you will find caries around and beneath it.

This page and the next five pages.

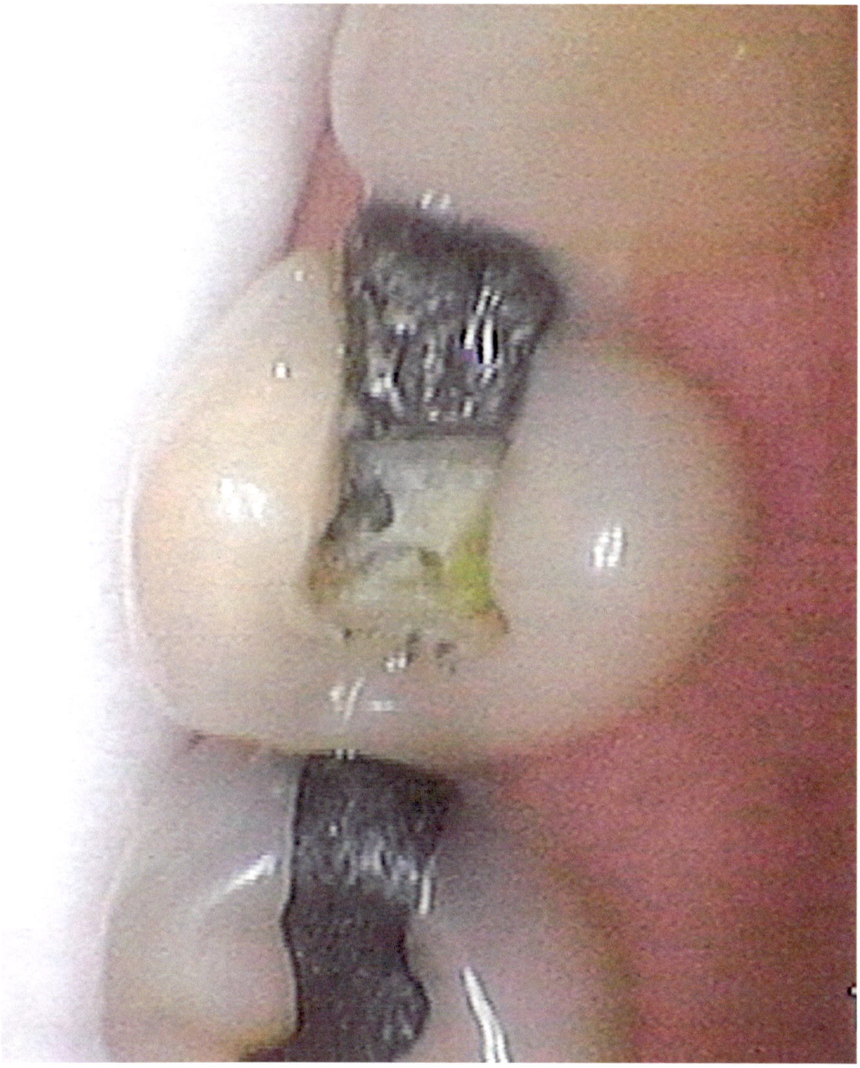

When you see this you know immediately that this tooth is in big trouble. In addition to listening to the patients symptoms, you need to percuss, push buccal → palatal, palpate the buccal sulcus. Take bitewing and periapical radiographs. Warn of the need for endodontic treatment or extraction. If patient wants to keep the tooth, get moving as you need every second of the appointment time that remains.

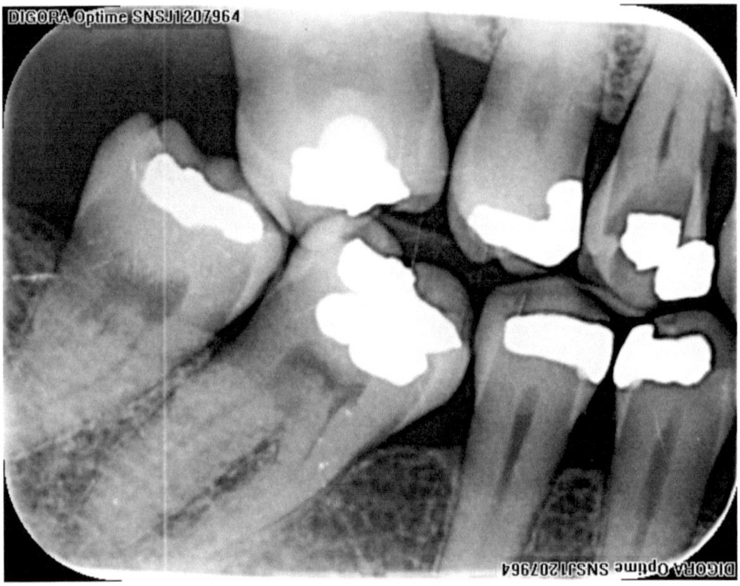


14MO amalgam filling has broken and the occlusal portion has sunk up into the mushy deep caries.

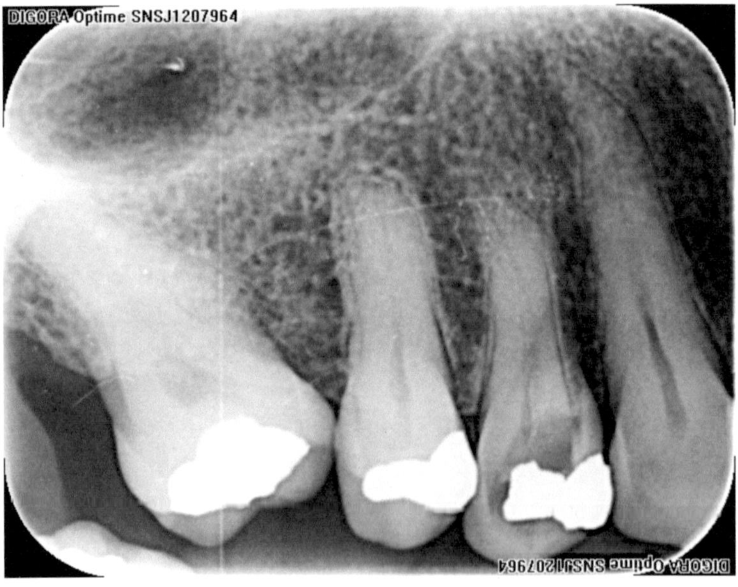


No periapical pathology seen in 14.

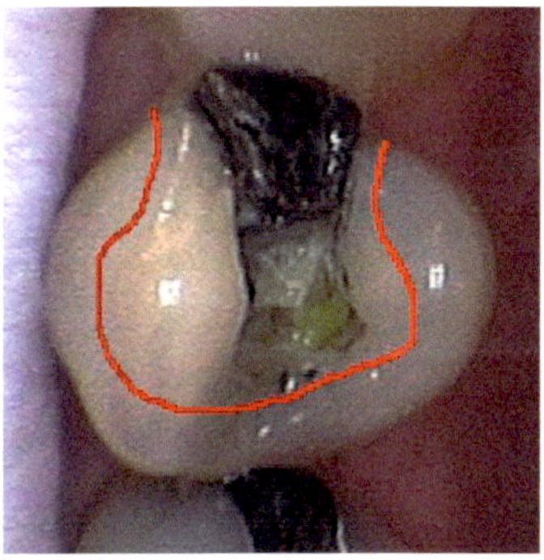

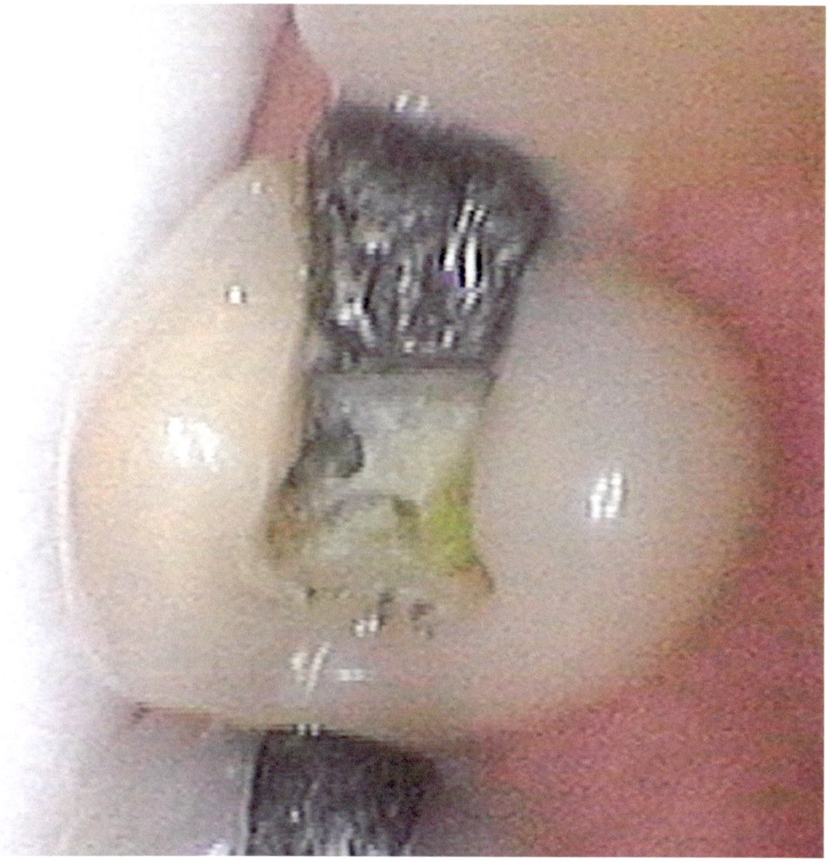

The light or cream colour tells you that this is rapidly spreading caries.

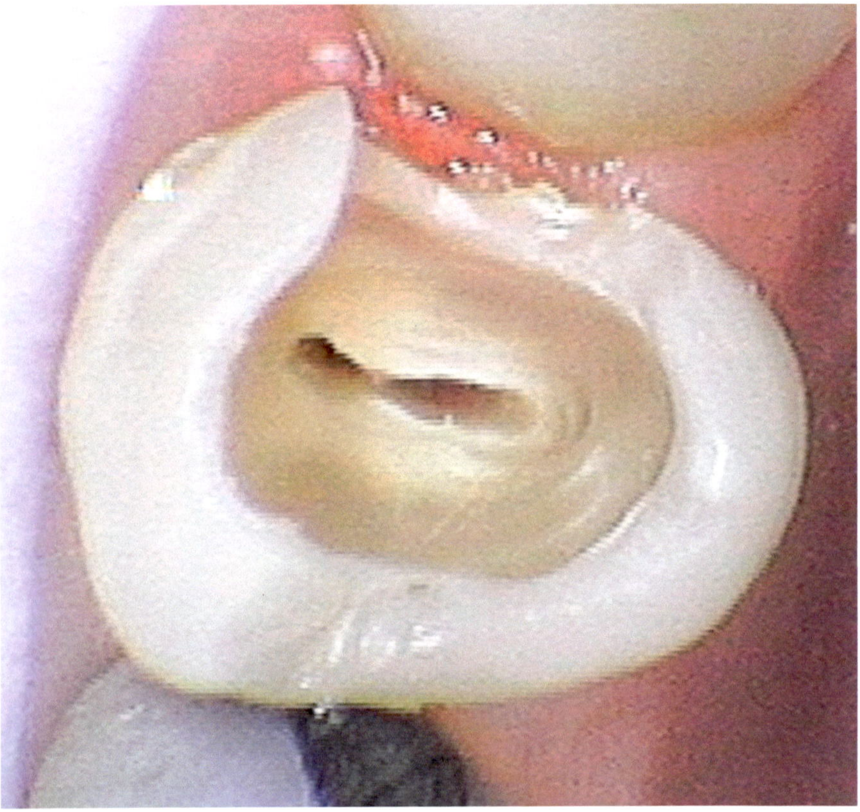

And sure enough, as expected, the caries was well into the pulp. You did well to advise the patient BEFOREHAND that this might happen.

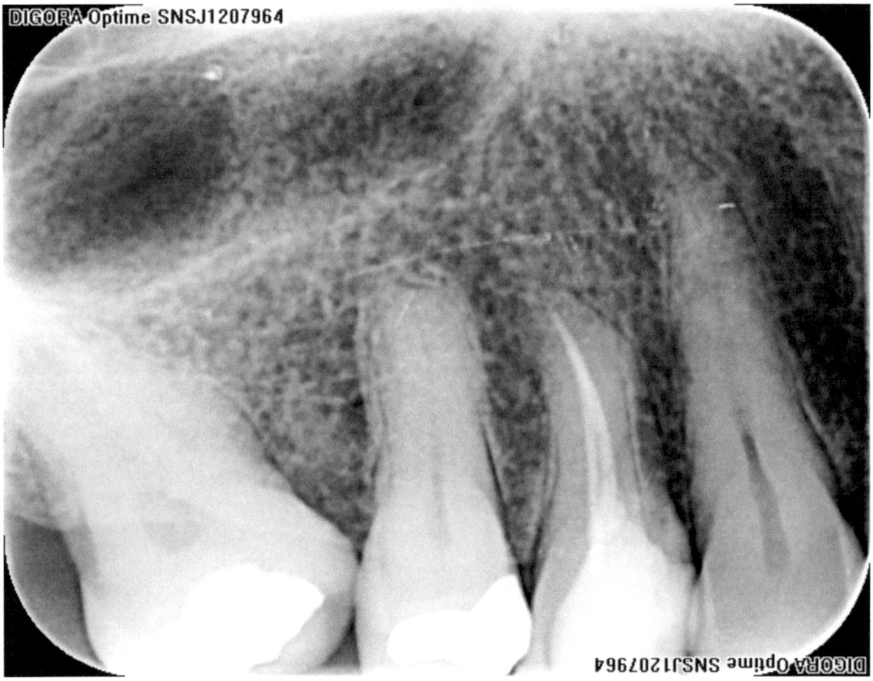


The tooth root filled and restored.

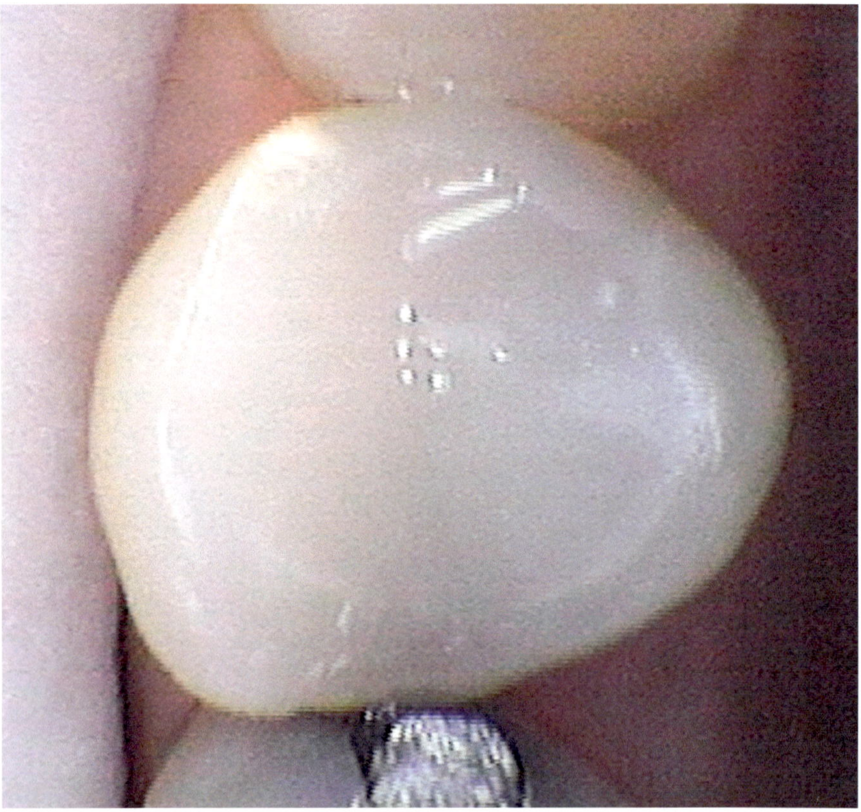

Final filling in 14MO – compared to tooth at presentation, page 123.

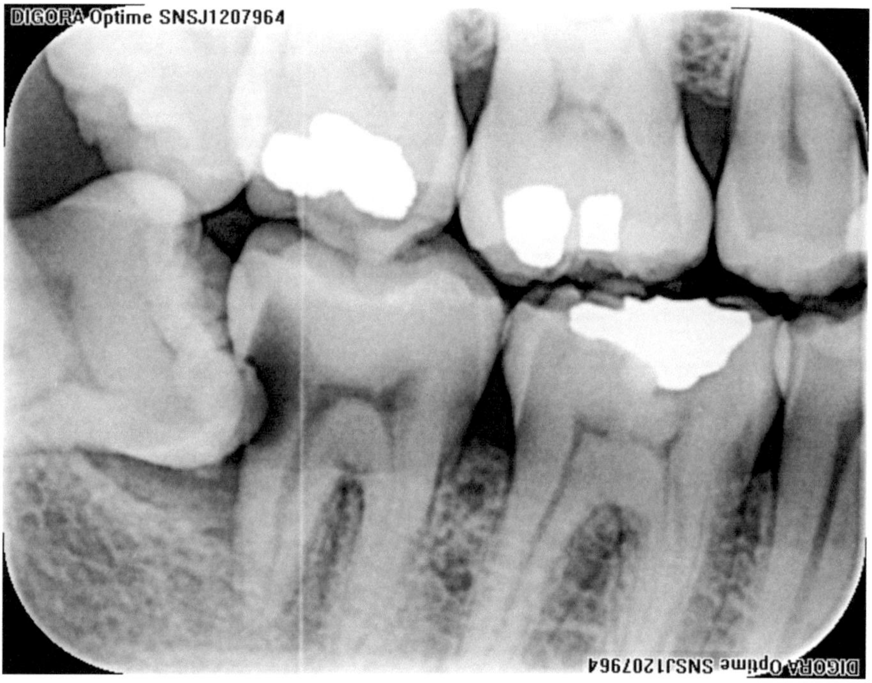


Generally 95% of the time a partly erupted mesioangularly impacted 8 will cause caries low down on the distal of the 7. You would be doing the patient a disservice by not removing the 8 early.

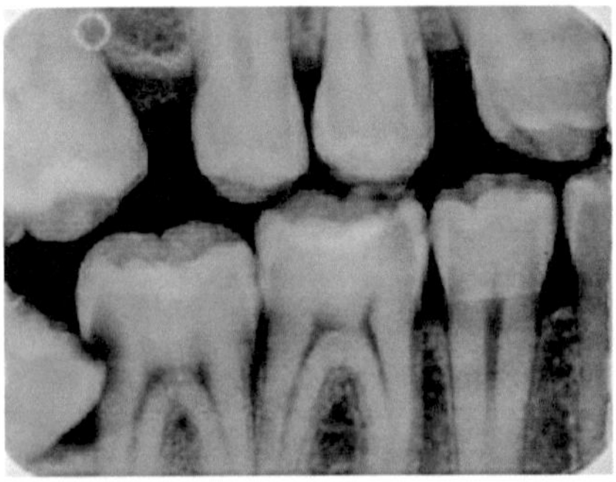

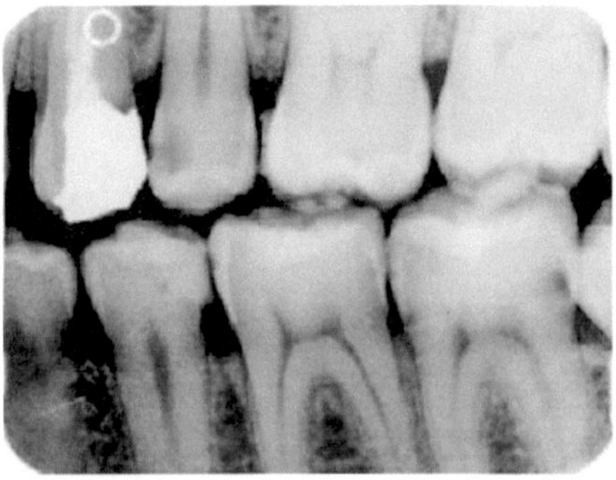

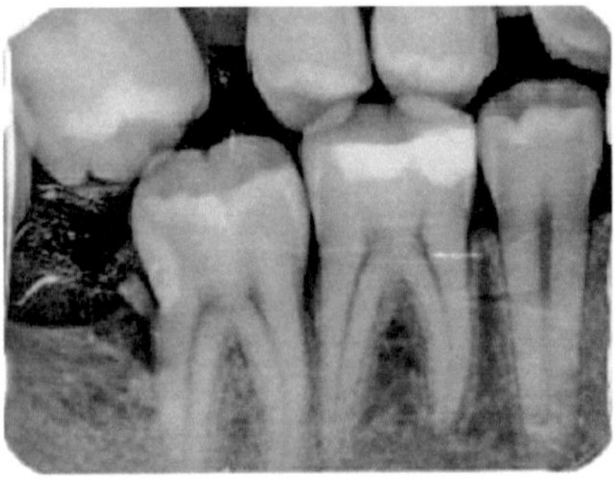

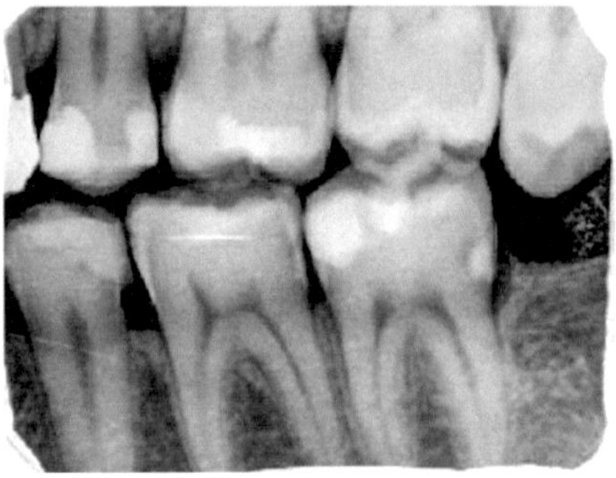

The mesio-angularly impacted 38 and 48 have contributed to dental caries in 37D and 47D. Ideally wait 6 weeks after the removal of 38 and 48 to allow for tissue healing and contraction to take place in the sockets before you attend to the distal caries in the second molars.

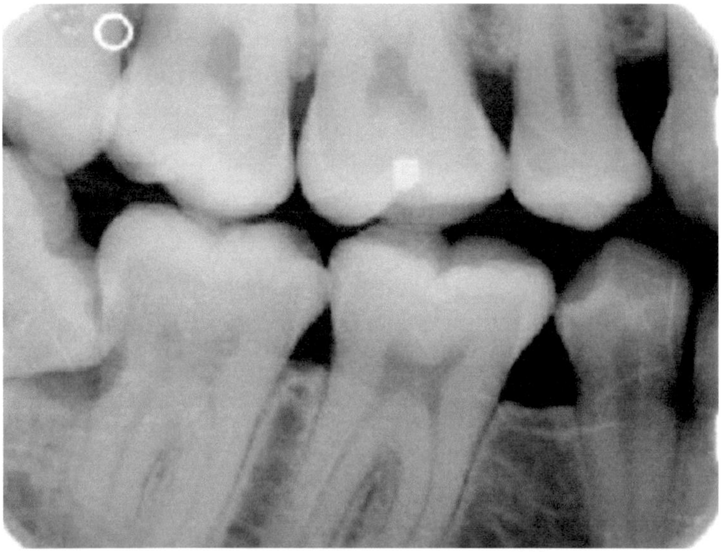

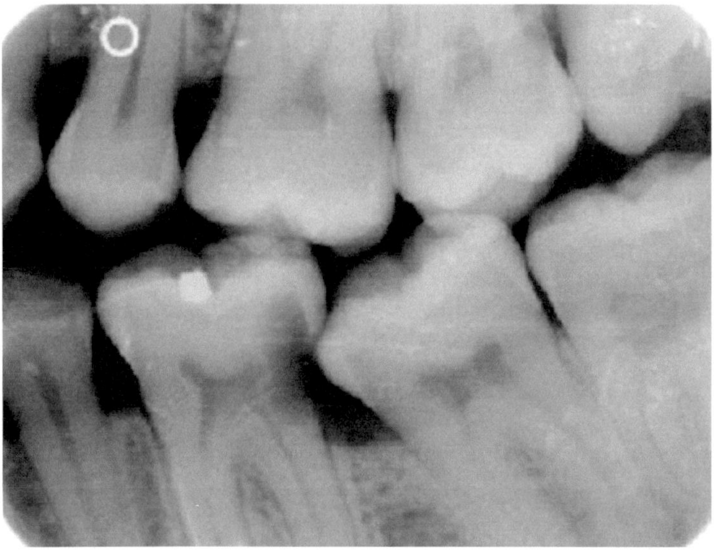

In this case the mesio-angularly impacted 48 has led to caries in 47D. Note also that the mesio-angularly impacted 37 has done the same thing to 36D. (36 quite likely will require endodontic care).

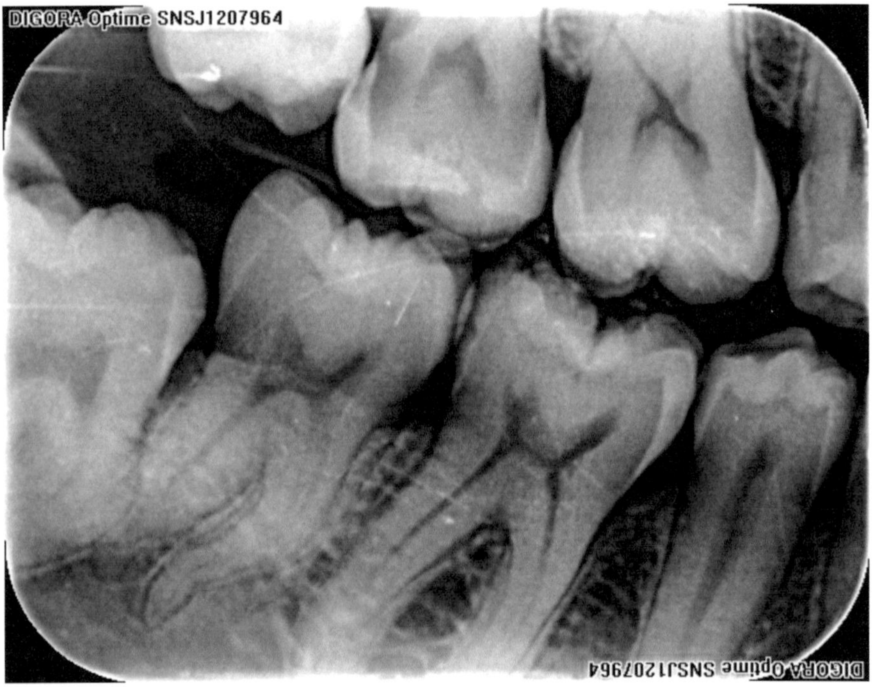


Deep caries 17 distal as a result of the 18 being mesio-angularly impacted into it.

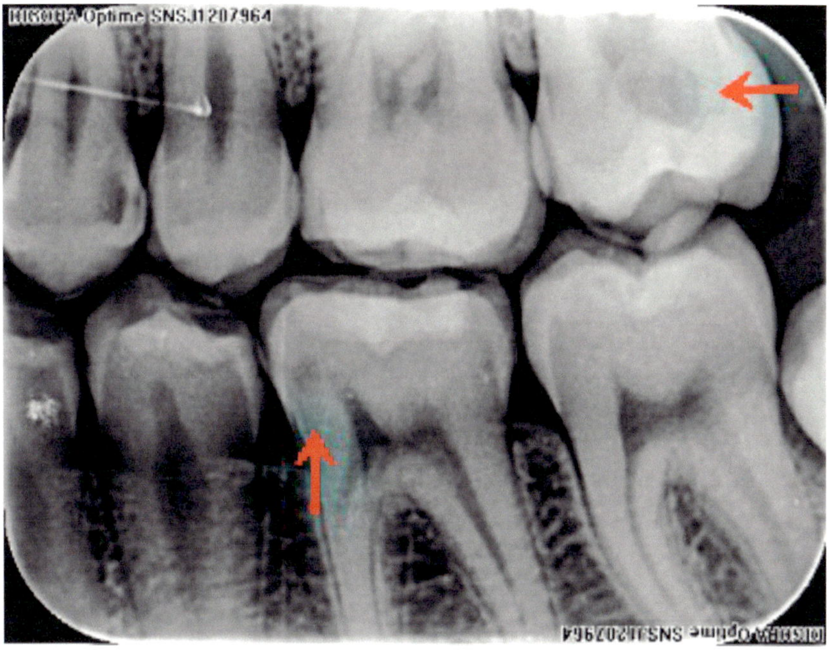

Look at the radiolucency 36MB area. The mesial enamel is intact. This is a cavity in the buccal aspect. 27 has a deep buccal cavity.

# Cemental
# CARIES

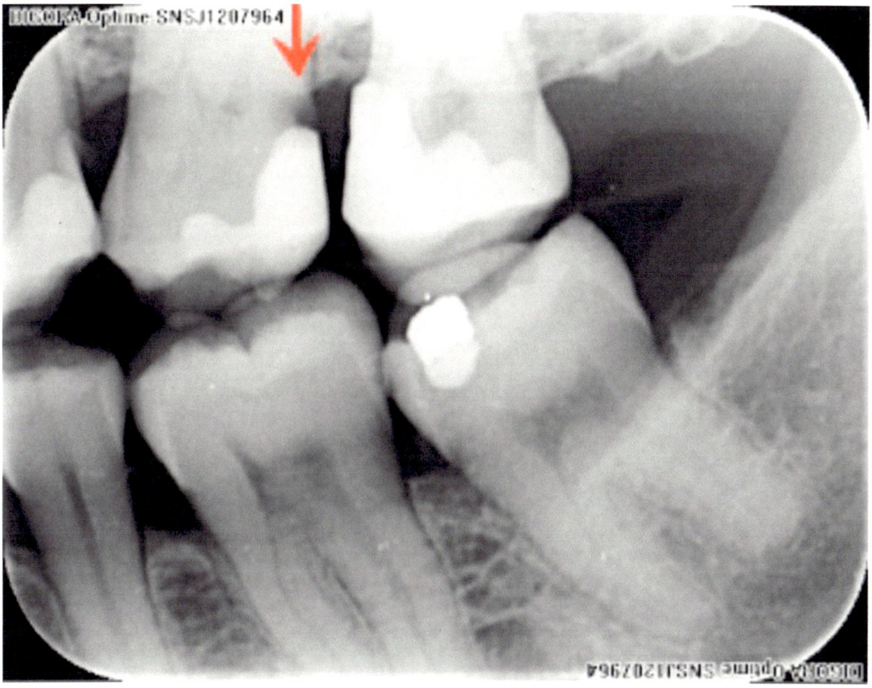


Cervical and subgingival caries 26D – a challenge, so take your time. Leave the patient better off, not worse off.

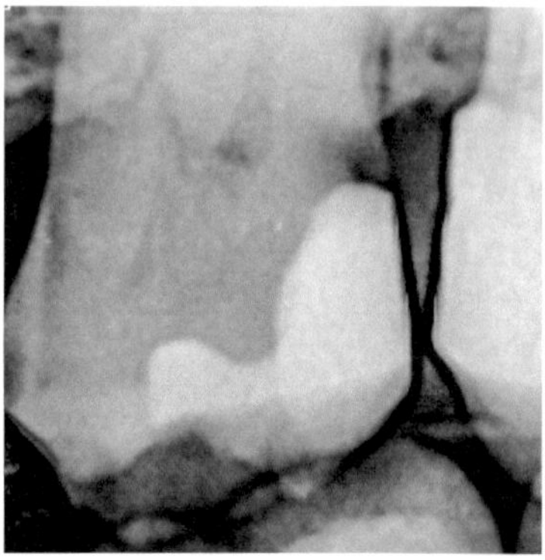

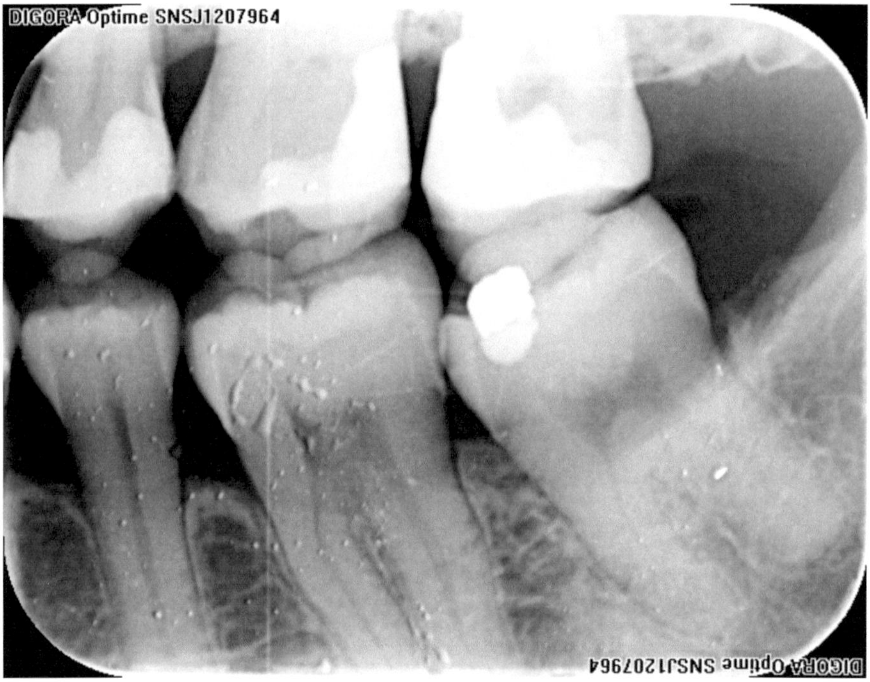


26 distal cemental caries removed and the tooth restored.

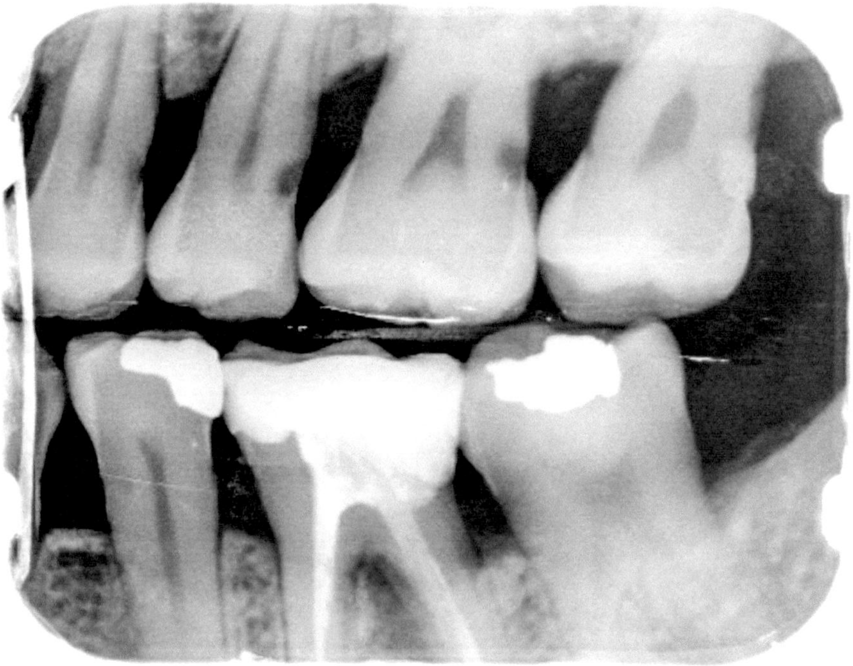

Root caries, particularly, presents a challenge. You will encounter it more as patients live longer, keep their teeth for longer and, sadly, get to situations when they cannot care for their teeth as before. Look at the caries high up on 24D, 25D and 26D.

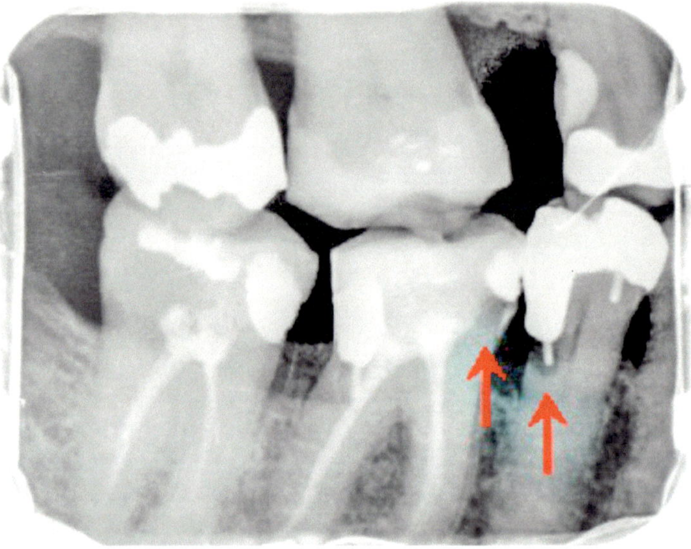

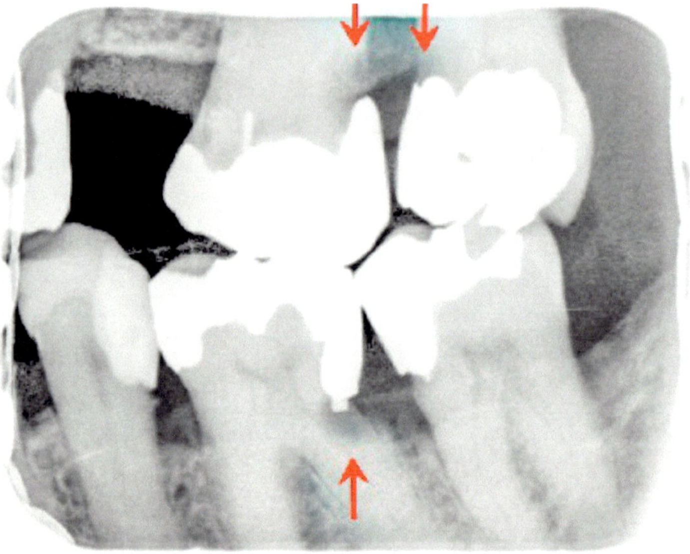

So, so very sad when the elderly and infirm can now no longer look after themselves, with deep cervical interproximal problems arising. Deep caries in 26D, 27M, 45D, 46M and 36D.

36 and 45 present a huge challenge.

From this

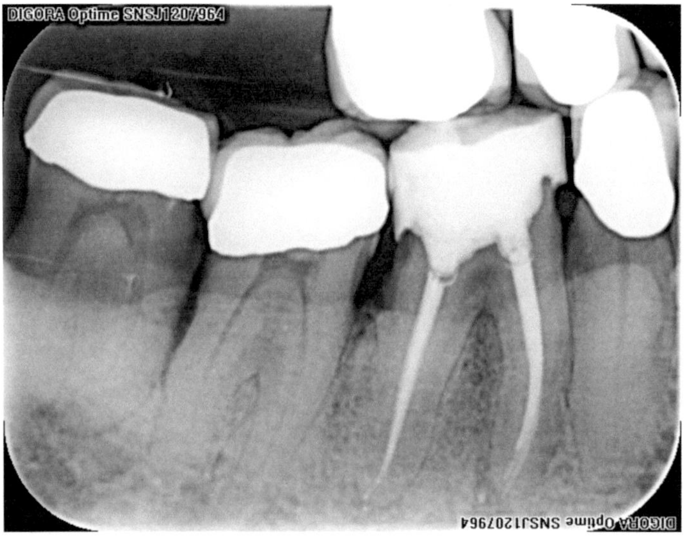


To this

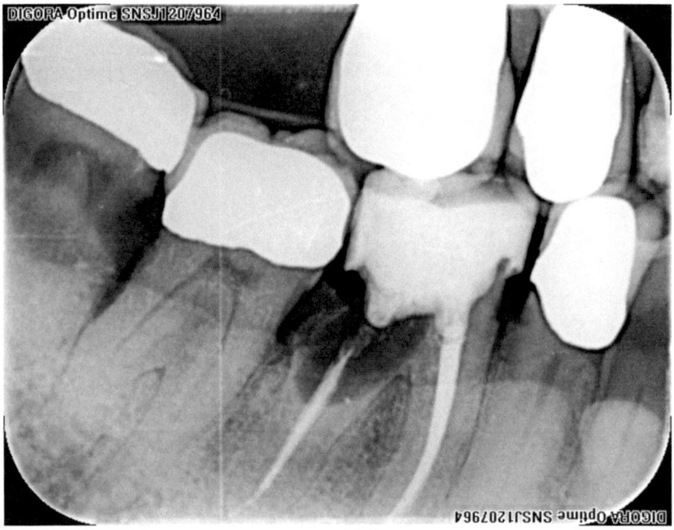


in less than 3 years.

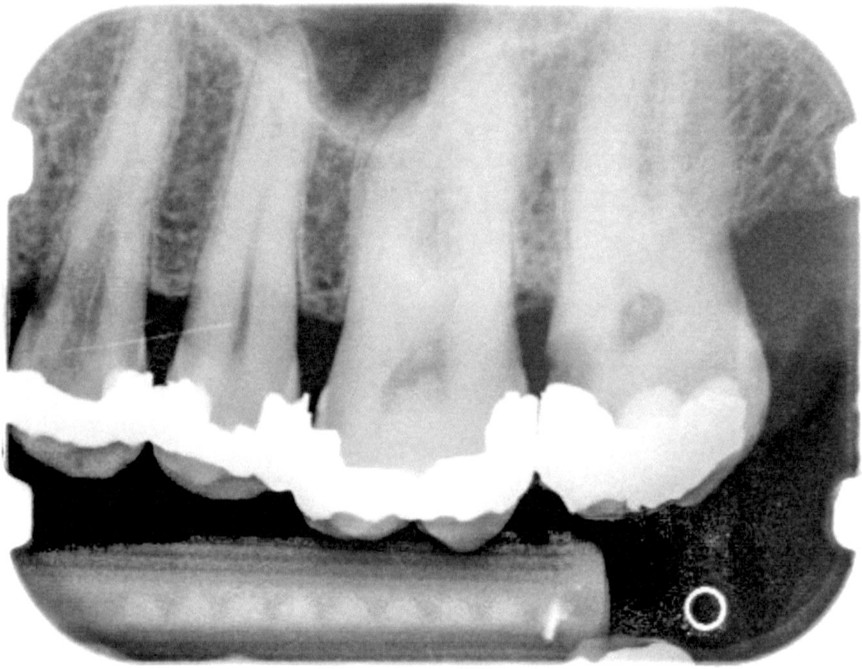

Deep caries 27M, but see the unusual appearance of 24.

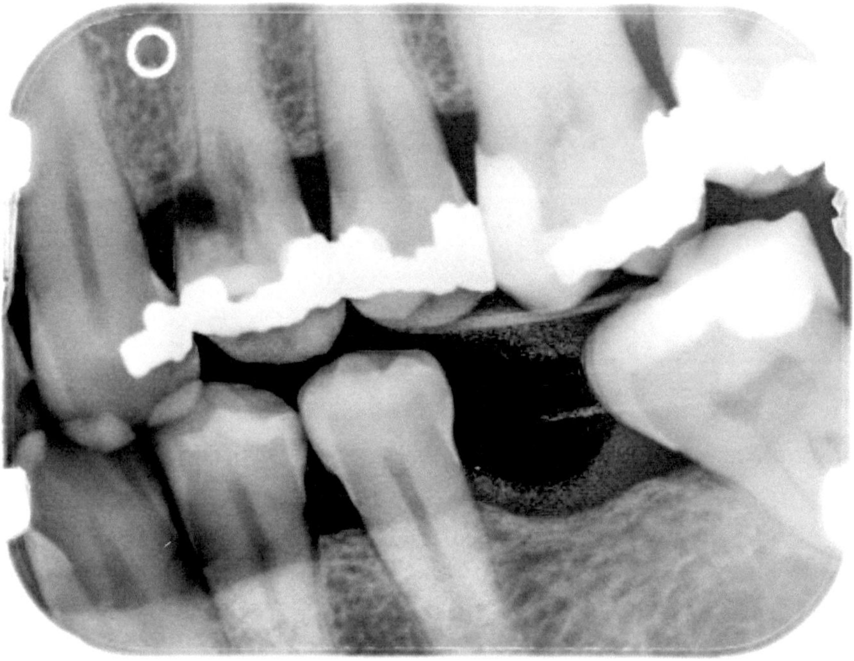

24M exhibits cervical external invasive resorption.

# *Time to*
# GET YOU THINKING

This page and the next four pages.

June 2013

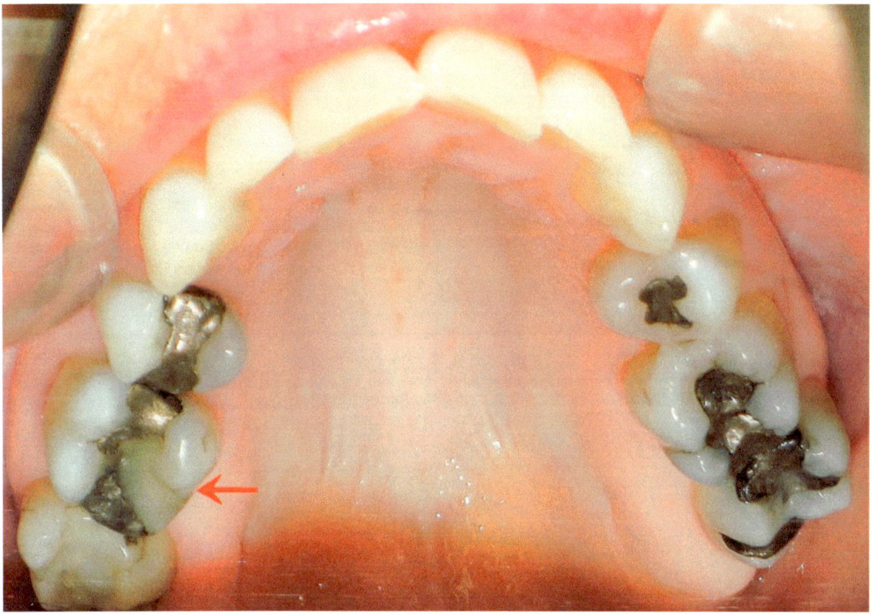

A 60 year old patient with many large old amalgam fillings.

17 has a composite resin filling.

16 has suffered a fracture to DP cusp and has had a resin filling repair to this area.

Clean teeth, healthy gingivae.

June 2013

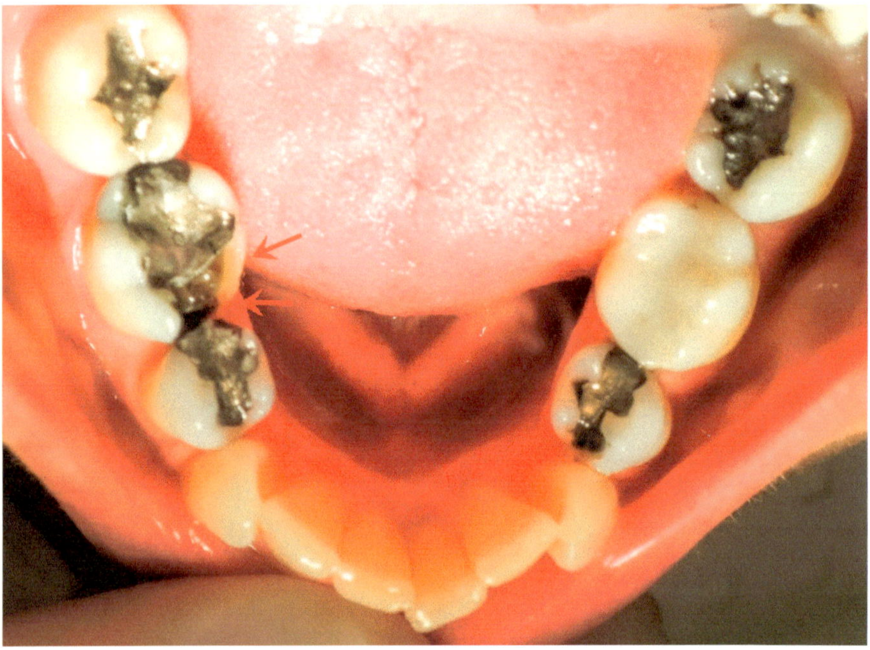

The lower arch of the same patient, many large old amalgam fillings.

36 has had breakdown and now has a large MOL composite resin filling.

46 has a wide filling, the ML cusp has broken away and the MO part of the amalgam has broken off. Patient wants a repair/"patch" to MOL corner.

February 2011

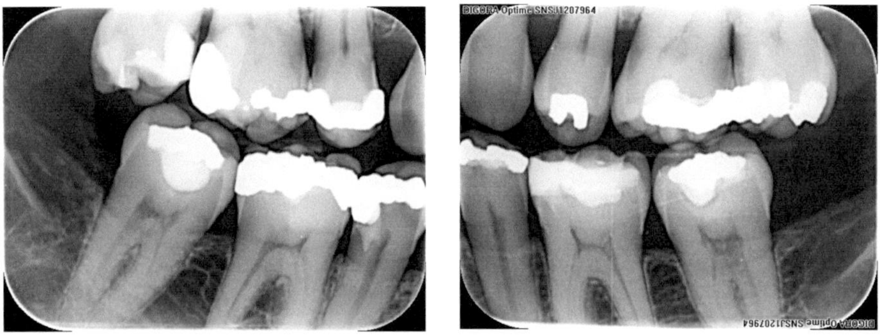

June 2013

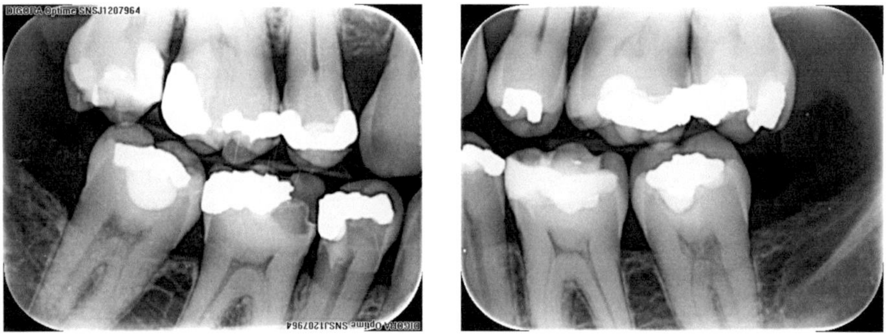

Heavily filled teeth. This patient is stable, with breakdown of 46MOL only. The bone health is good.

February 2018

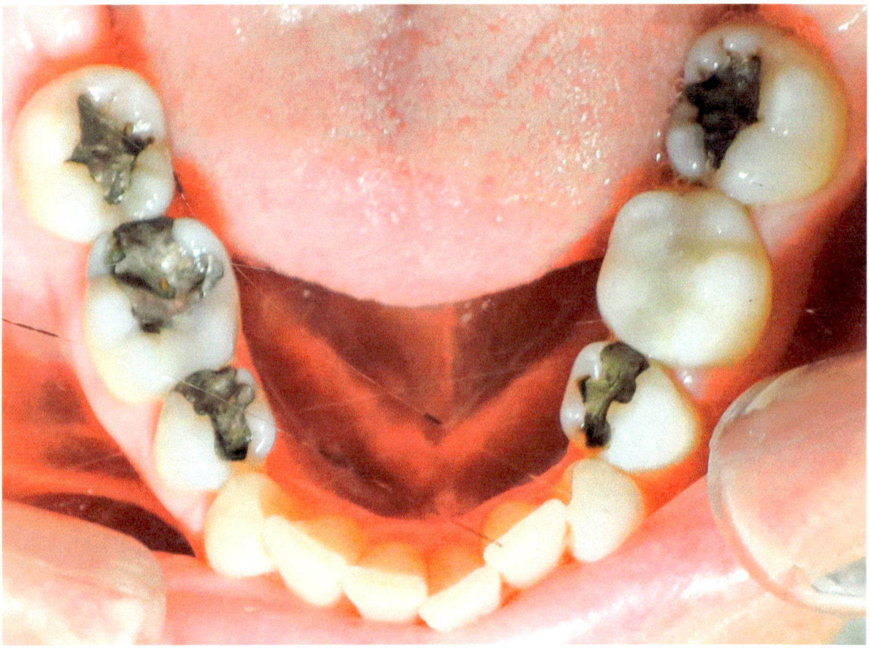

46 seen with its MOL composite resin repair 4¾ years later.

No changes / breakdown elsewhere.

Ideally crown 36 and 46 but patient does not want this.

Not everyone wants, or can afford, the ideal.

Basic dentistry, done well, can last.

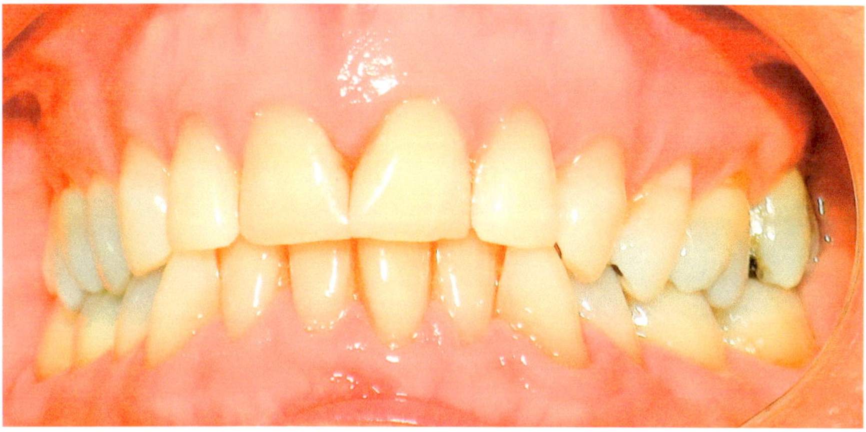

Immaculate oral hygiene, has not had a scale and polish for two years. Note the excellent gingival health. This patient is stable except for one variable, that being that because she has had so many large fillings placed in the past, there will inevitably be breakdown. This has happened on 16, 36 and 46 as you have seen.

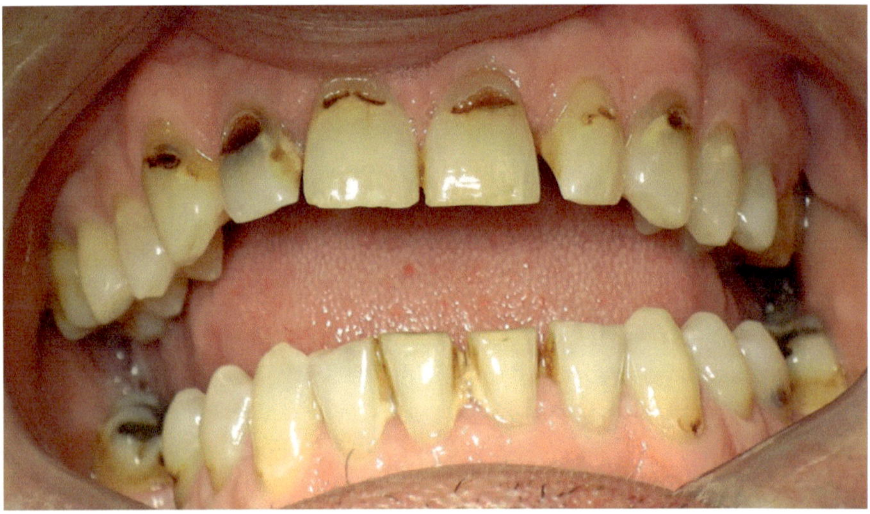

Some active caries 12L and 23B. From a strictly caries perspective, nothing else has to be done, aesthetics aside.

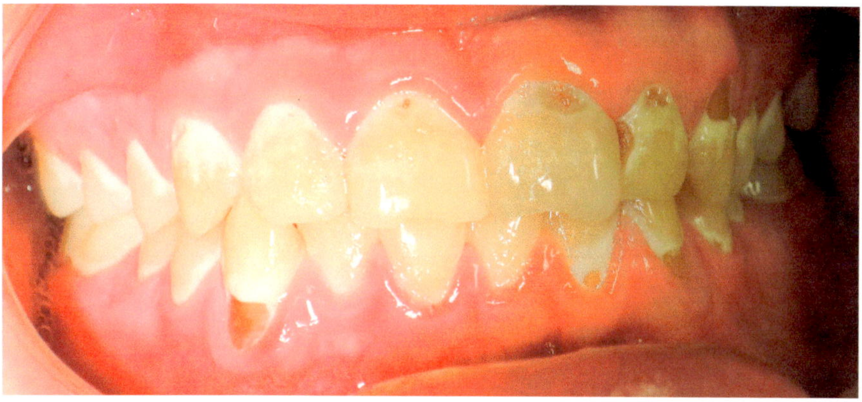

Extensive breakdown.

Lots of decalcification.

Fillings alone of no use unless causative factors are eliminated.

Tooth brushing instruction, optimising oral hygiene, flossing.

Dietary analysis, saliva flow and composition check.

Use of Colgate Neutrafluor 5000 and Tooth Mousse in trays.

Resin infiltration later.

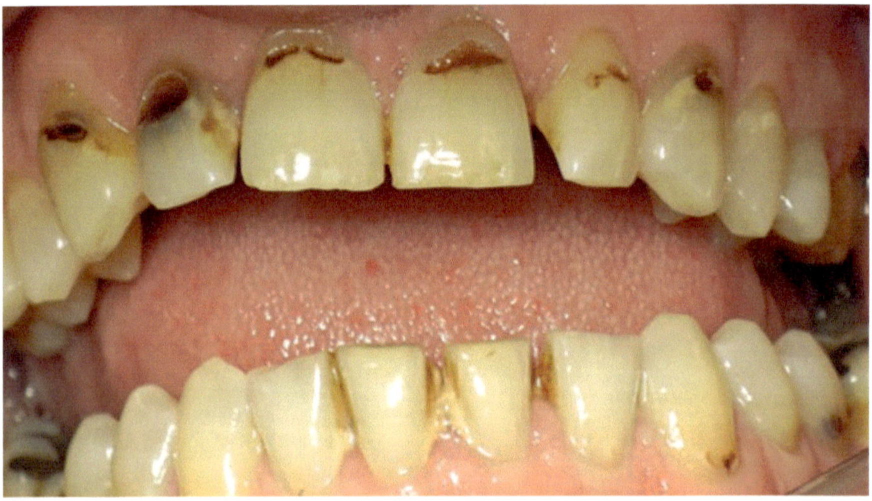

Most teeth have arrested caries. A stable mouth.

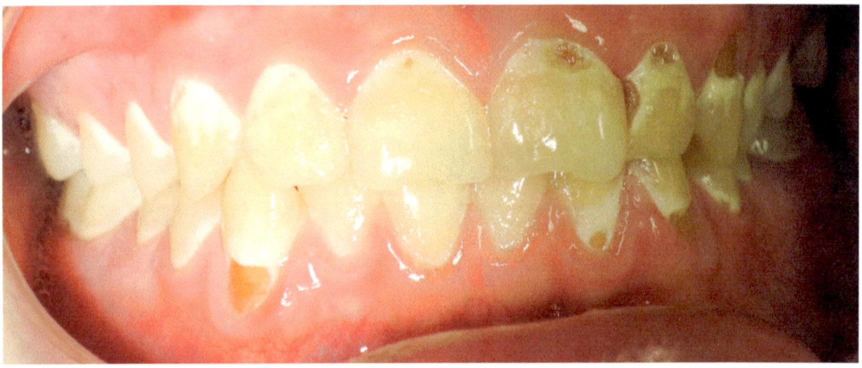

All teeth have extensive decalcification. A very unstable mouth.

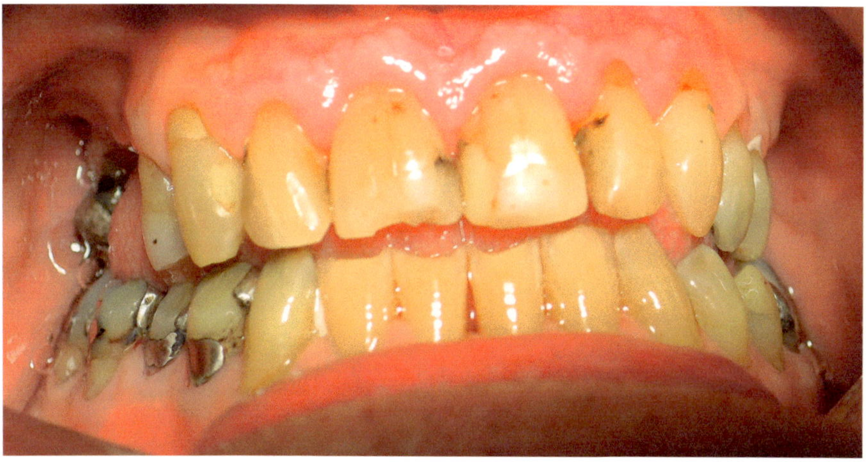

Evidently an elderly patient, worn lower incisor tips, lots of fillings, some worn. Staining at filling-tooth junctions.

No caries anywhere.

Only presented because had broken away the buccal cusp of 14 that had an existing old MOD amalgam filling.

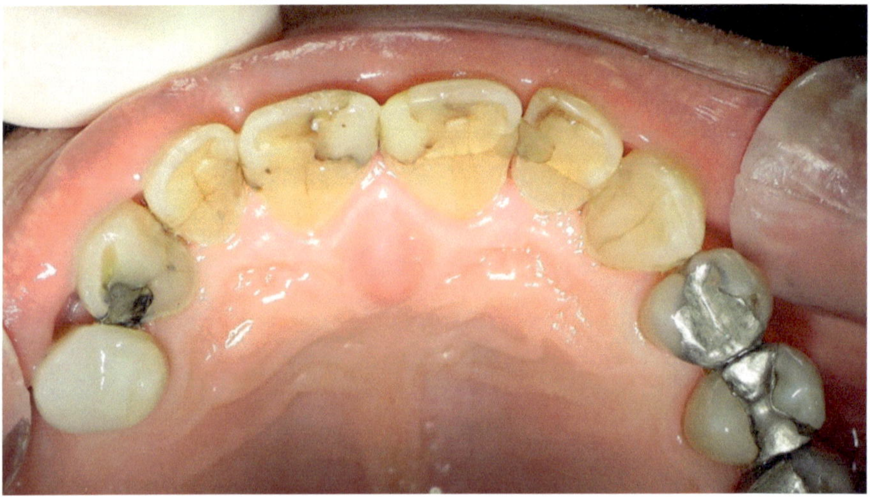

Fillings are old, many crack lines evident, no symptoms.

14 has been restored with a MODB resin restoration.

From a caries perspective, nothing else needs doing.

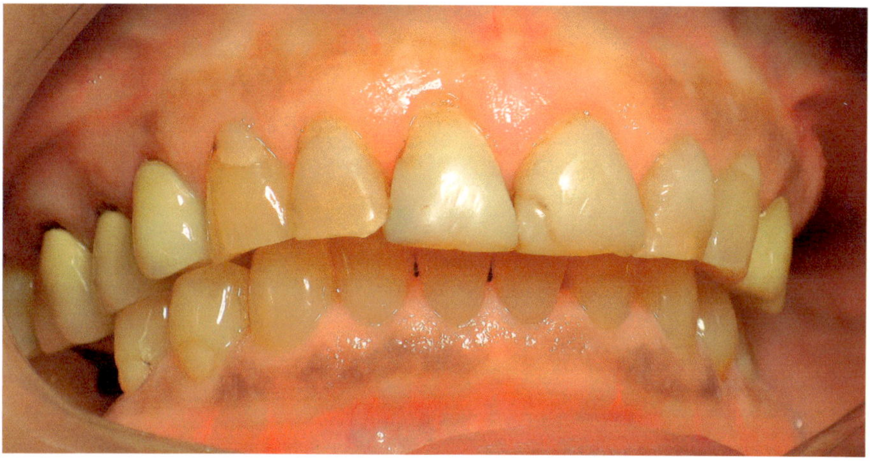

Some fillings are worn and look tatty.

The patient is happy and has no aesthetic concerns.

There is no caries and there is full function.

From a purely caries perspective, nothing needs to be done.

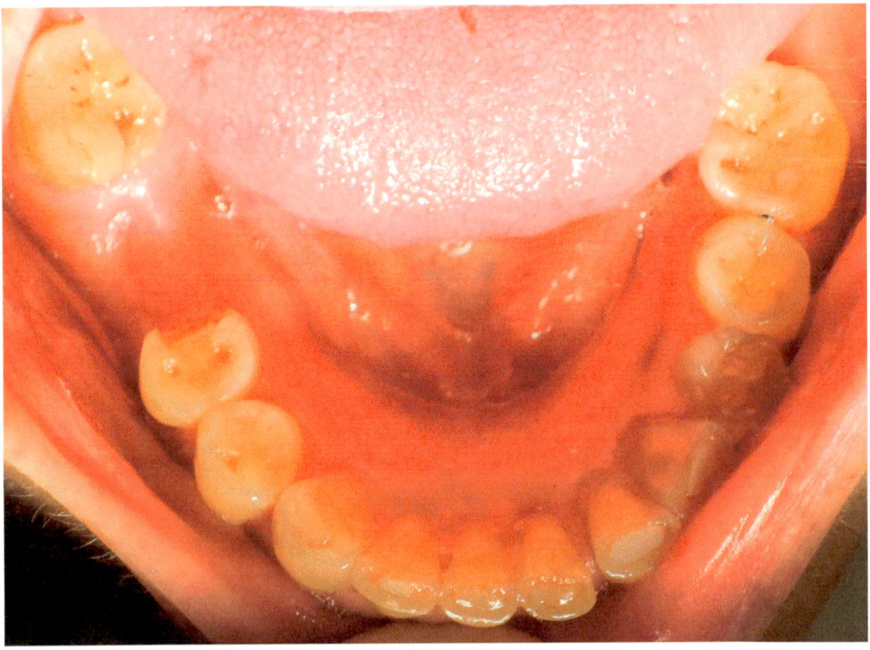

The same patient – lower arch.

You may want to fill 7 or 8 teeth, but again, from a purely caries perspective, you do not need to do a thing.

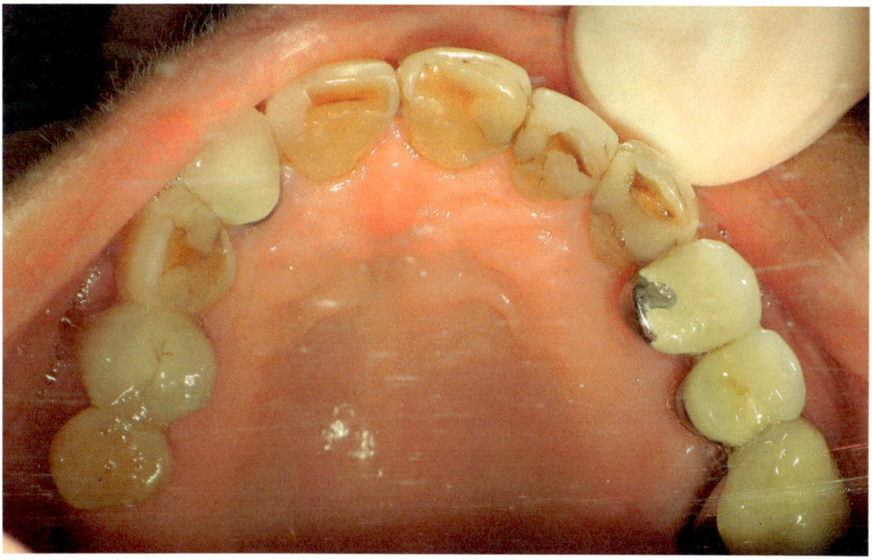

There is no caries in those upper anterior teeth.

Again, caries-wise you do not have to do a thing.

The teeth are heavily restored, there is evidence of strong chewing forces and erosion.

(We crowned 13, 11, 21, 22 and 23).

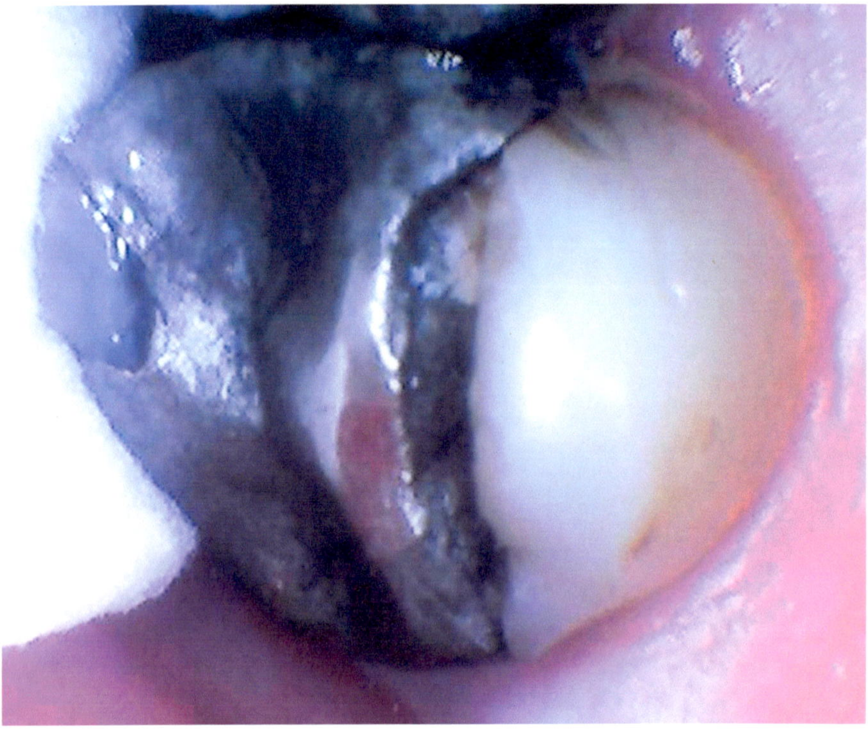

"Furrowing", or "ditching" at the amalgam/tooth interface from the loss of enamel prisms over many years.

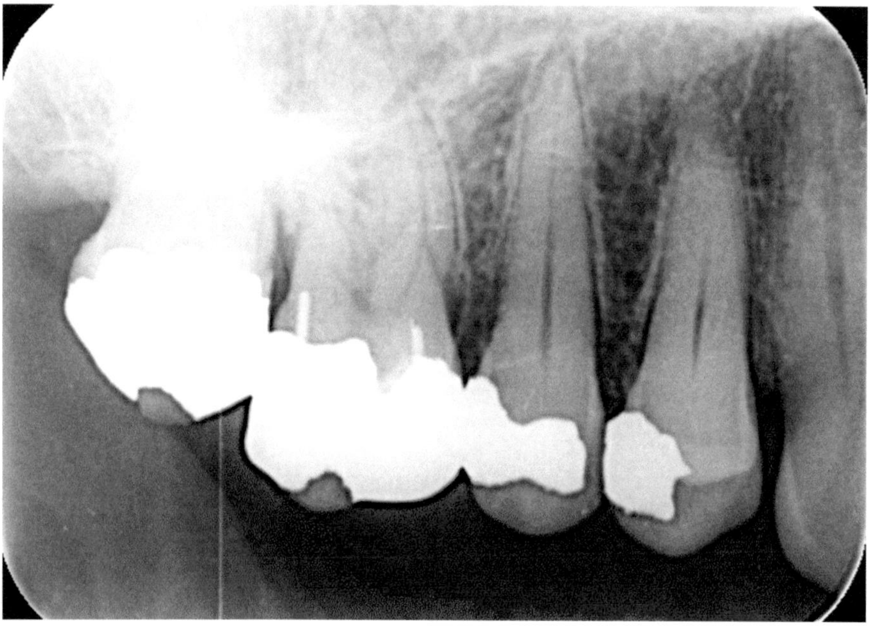

Tooth 17 as per previous page.

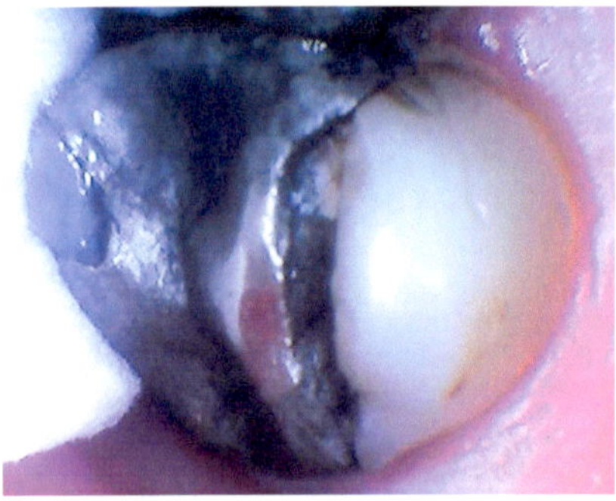

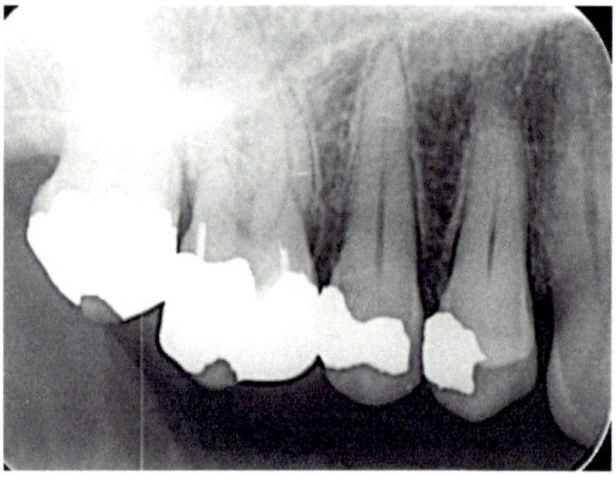

Before you get too clever, too drill happy and mutilate this tooth, consider:

This is an incidental finding, the patient has no symptoms.

The patient is 65 years old, this filling is maybe 40 years old.

"Ditching" occurs at an amalgam filling/enamel junction.

There is no caries. The filling is deep with a "base" on the roof of the pulp chamber.

Radiographically and clinically there is no detectable caries.

Could you tidy up the "ditch" and conservatively fill the groove with composite?

If you removed such a large old HUGELY SUCCESSFUL filling, can you do any better?

Will you end up having to root treat it and put a crown on?

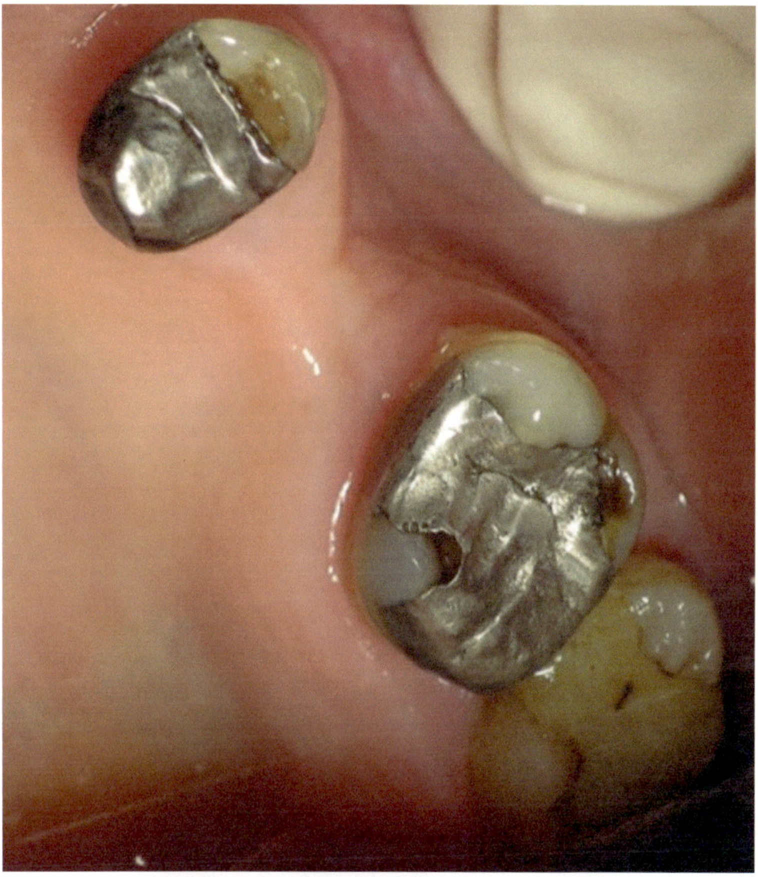

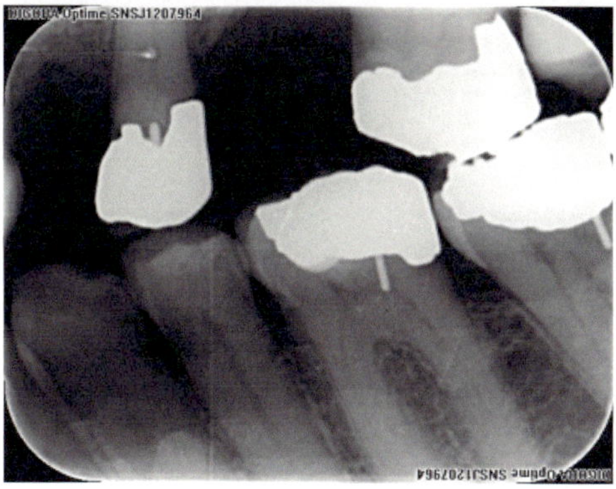

An elderly patient, good oral hygiene. Great gingival health. Large but old and successful amalgam fillings. No symptoms, no problems radiographically. Why do anything?

# *Potpourri*

# A FEW GENERAL CASES

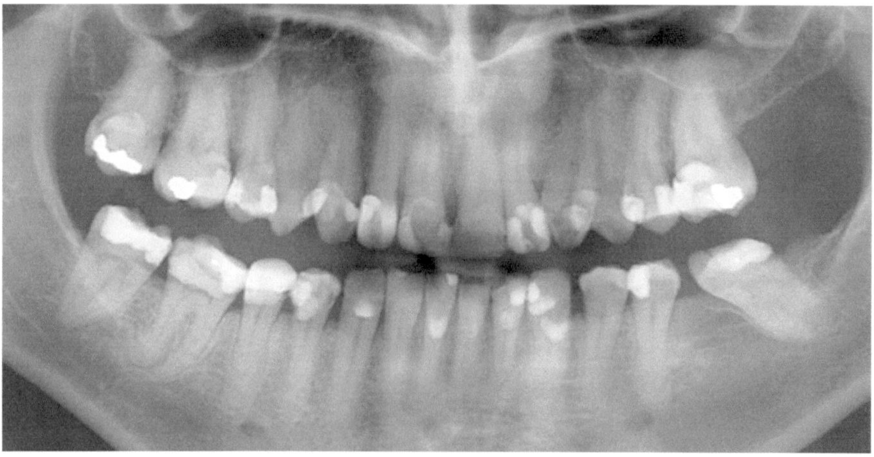

An OPG gives a good overview of mouth but is useless for fine detail on caries. You need bitewing radiographs for that. This patient has very heavily filled teeth. See next page.

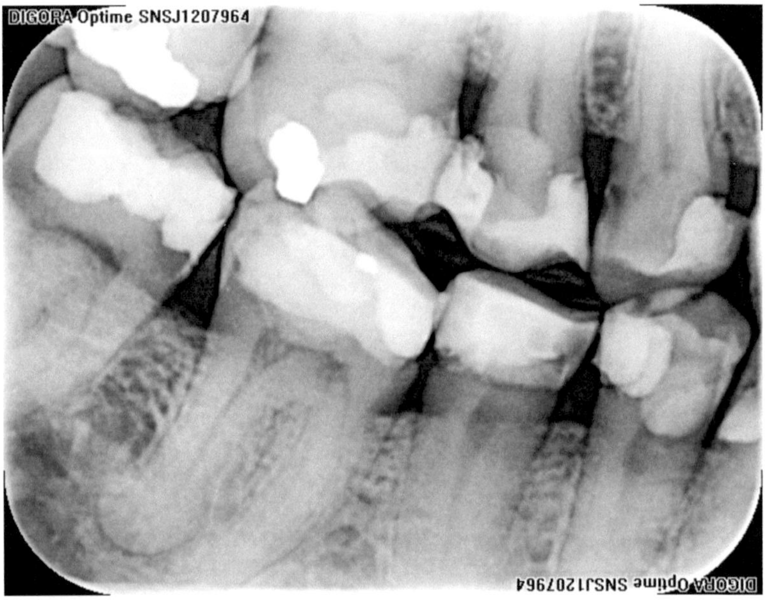


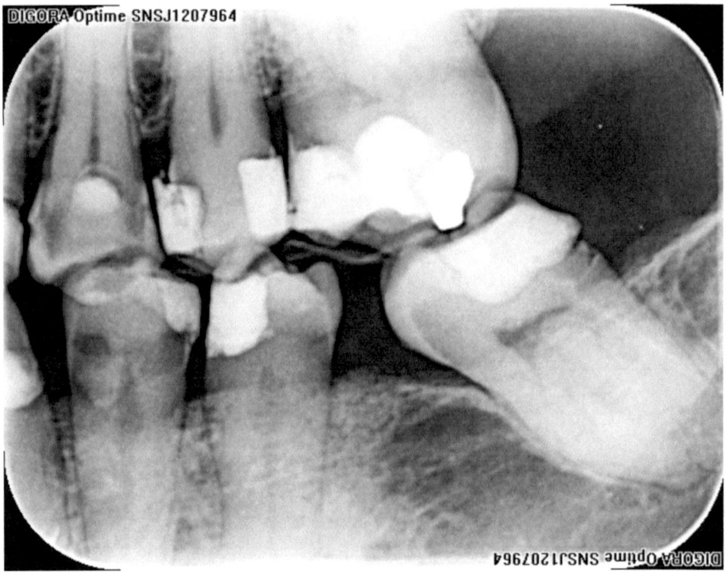


So tragic...... Where do you start? What if the patient cannot afford care? Do you continue with "patchwork"?

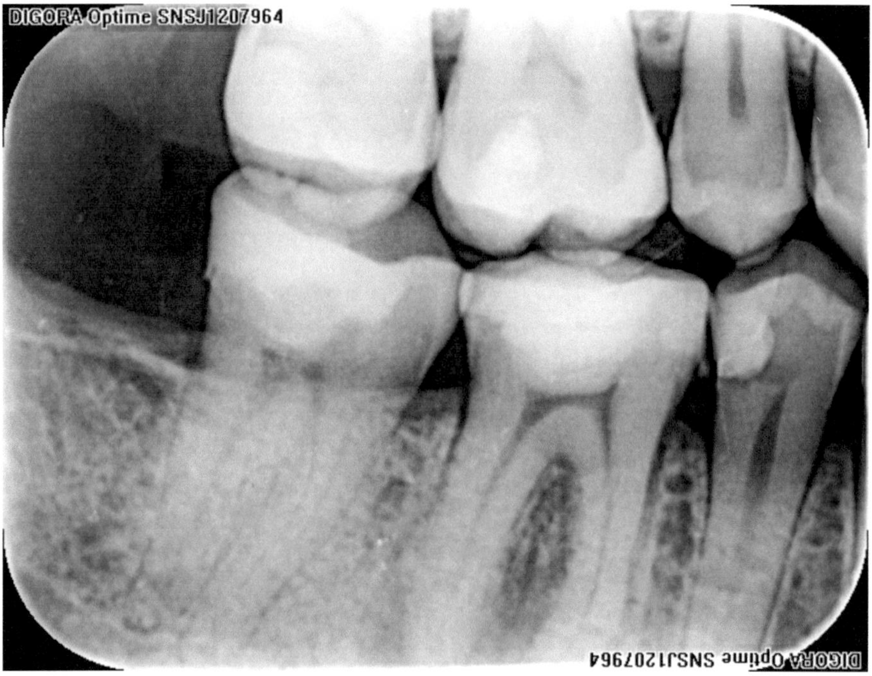


I mentioned earlier you must examine bitewing radiographs thoroughly.

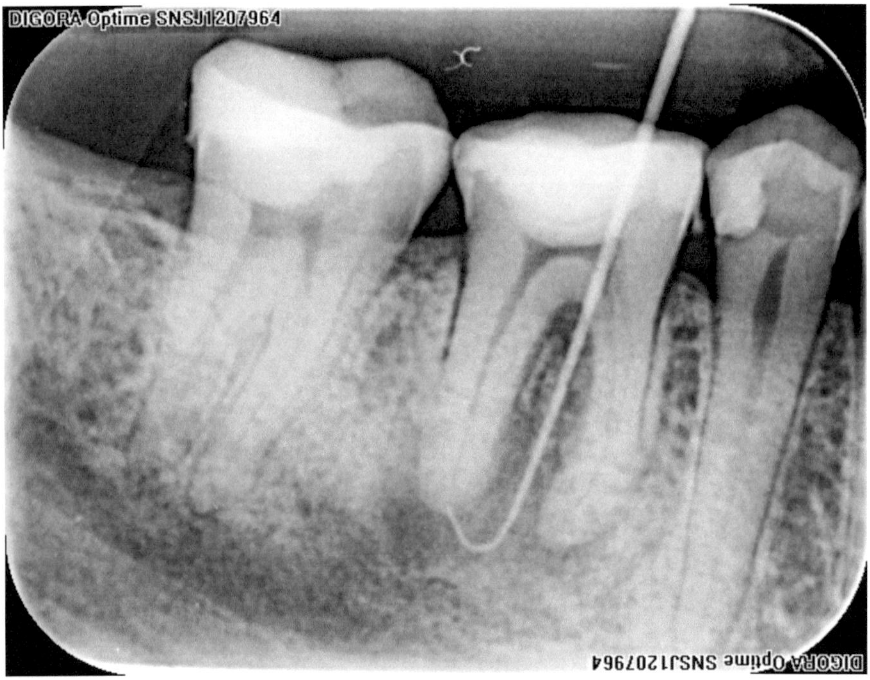


A symptom-free, chronically non-vital 46, discharging from a buccal sinus. Did you see a hint of the periapical lesion on the bitewing (previous page)?

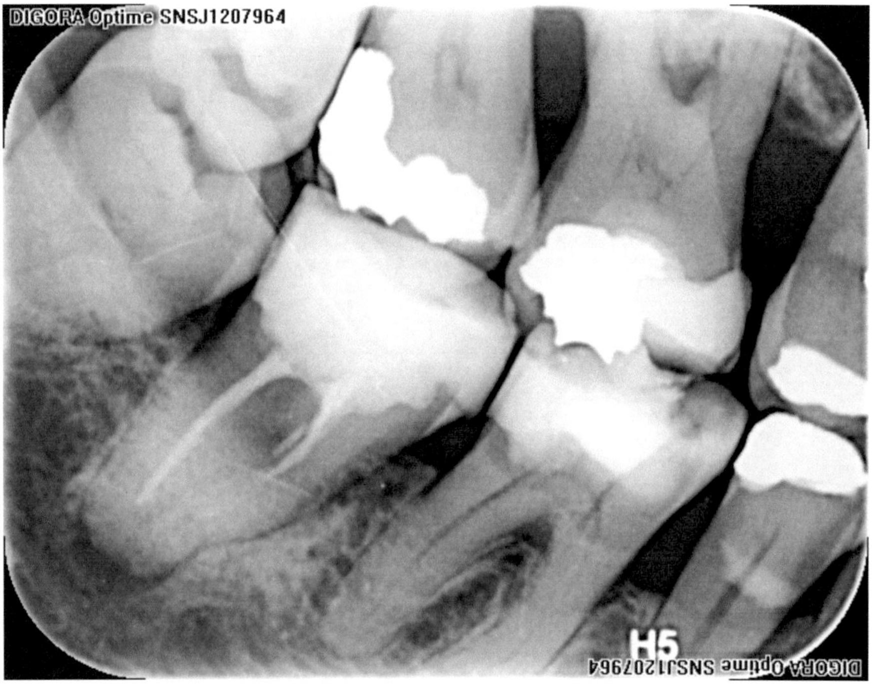


47 is poorly root filled and has associated periapical pathology.

46 has a large wide and deep buccal abrasion lesion.

Extensive alveolar bone loss 16 and 17.

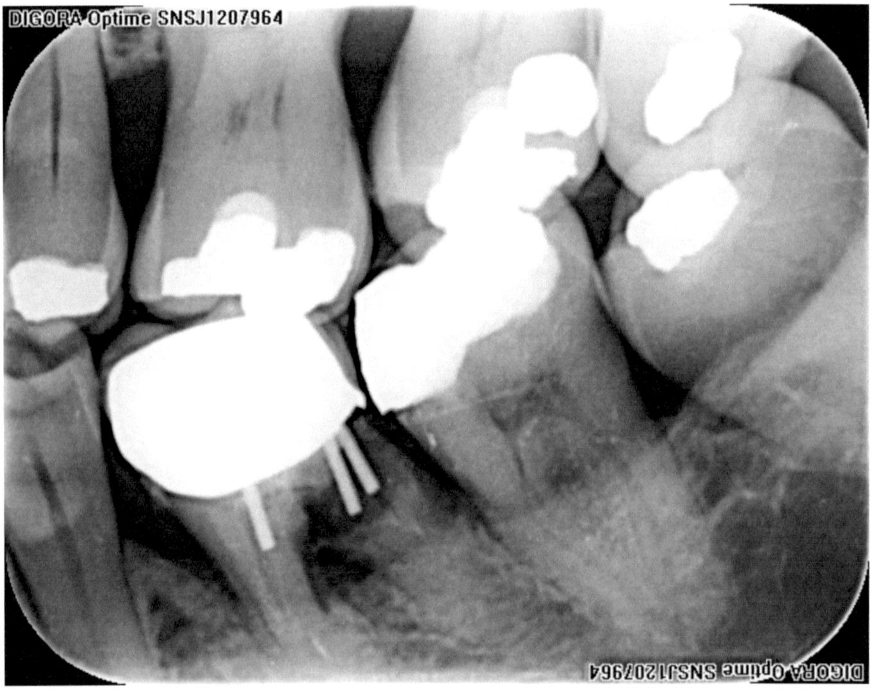


Extensive caries in 36 that has separated the distal root from the coronal aspect.

25-26-27 area shows alveolar bone loss.

This page and the next four pages.

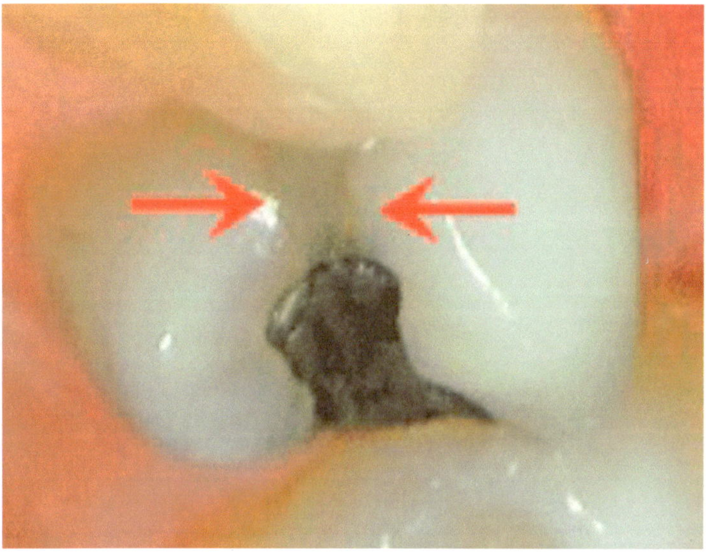

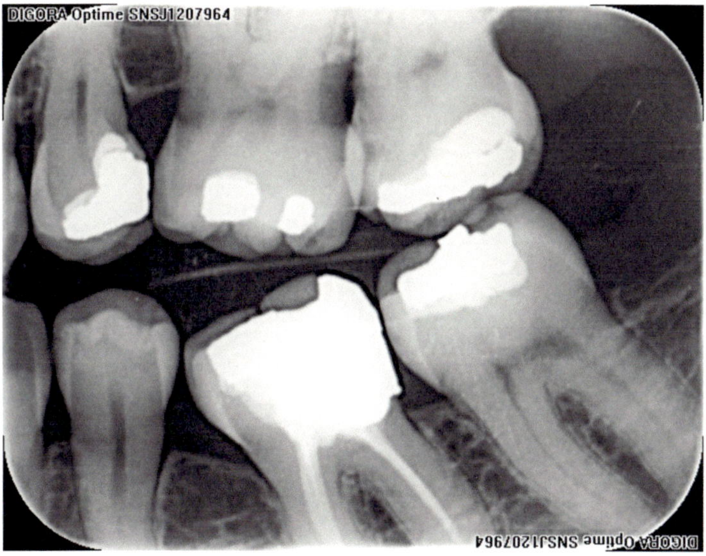


24 old disto-occlusal amalgam filling which is very deep and a crack is seen in the mesial marginal ridge.

A mesial to distal sagittal crack is suspected.

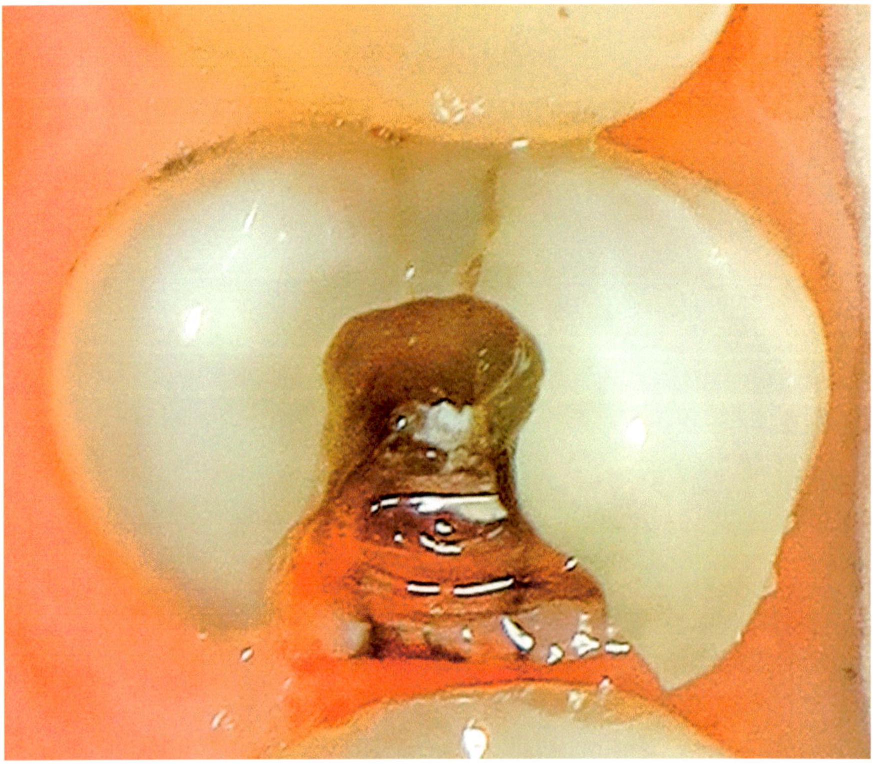

Upon removal of DO filling.

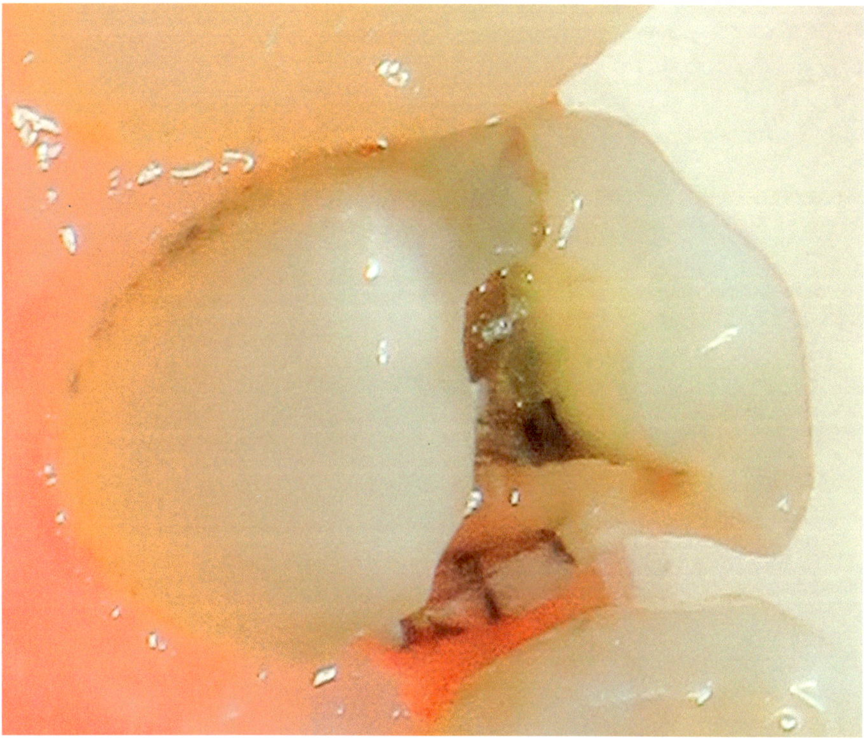

View from palatal aspect.

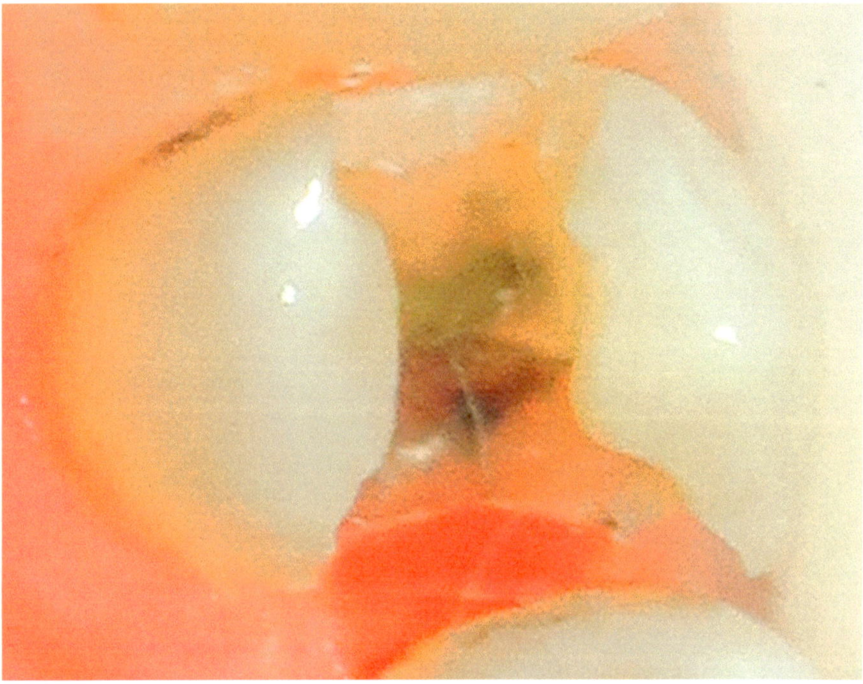

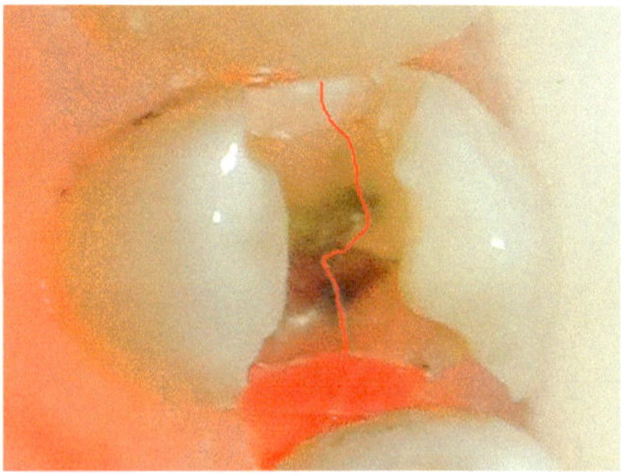

The fractured mesial marginal ridge removed. The cavity is caries-free.

A sagittal split is seen running mesial to distal.

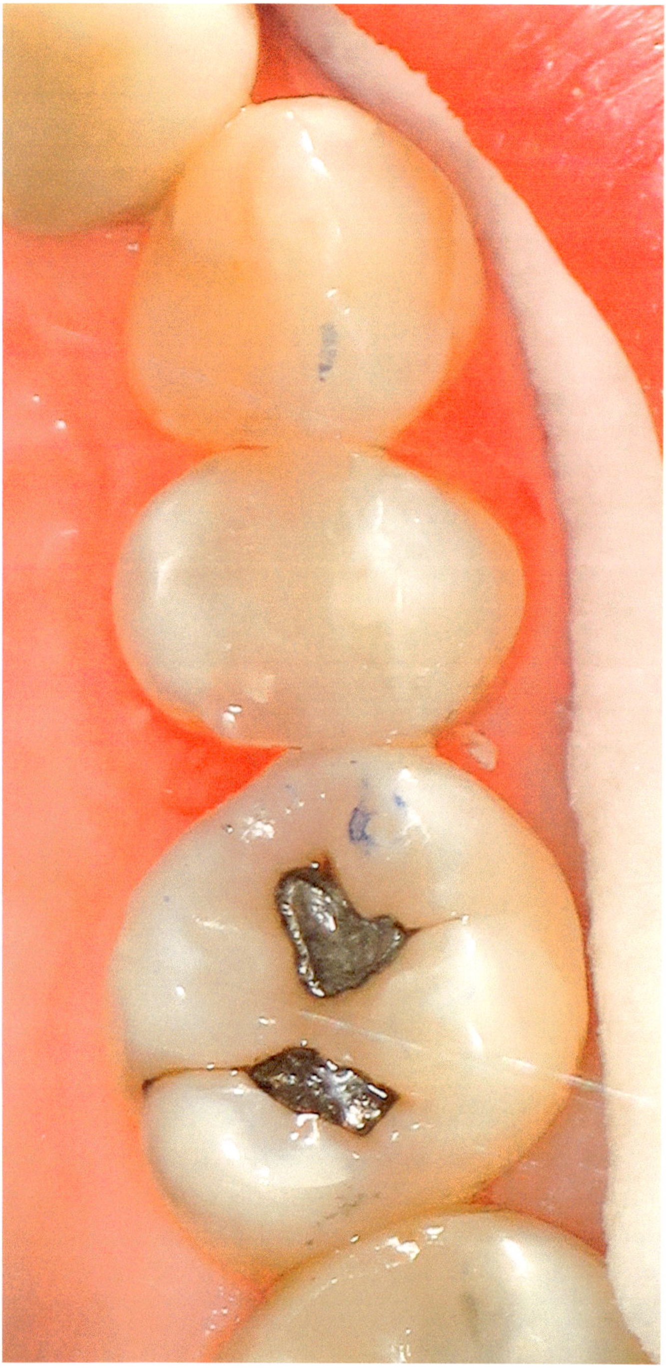

The tooth filled. Ideally requires a crown.

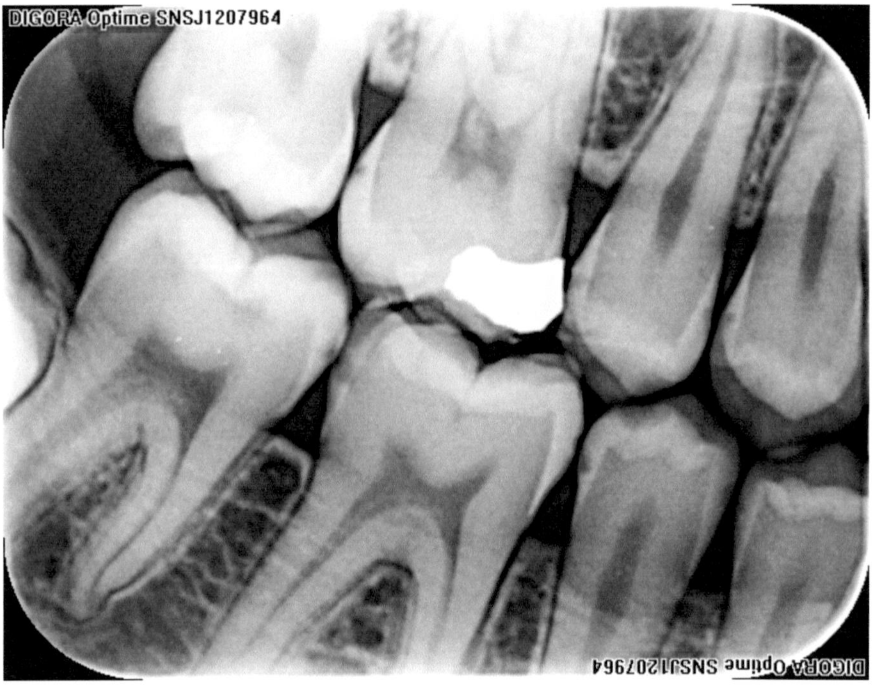


By now I hope you can differentiate between lesions in enamel only (to monitor), those where you have to intervene, and the borderline ones (15D,46D) where all other factors must be considered – oral hygiene, gingival health, does the patient floss, how stable is the mouth?

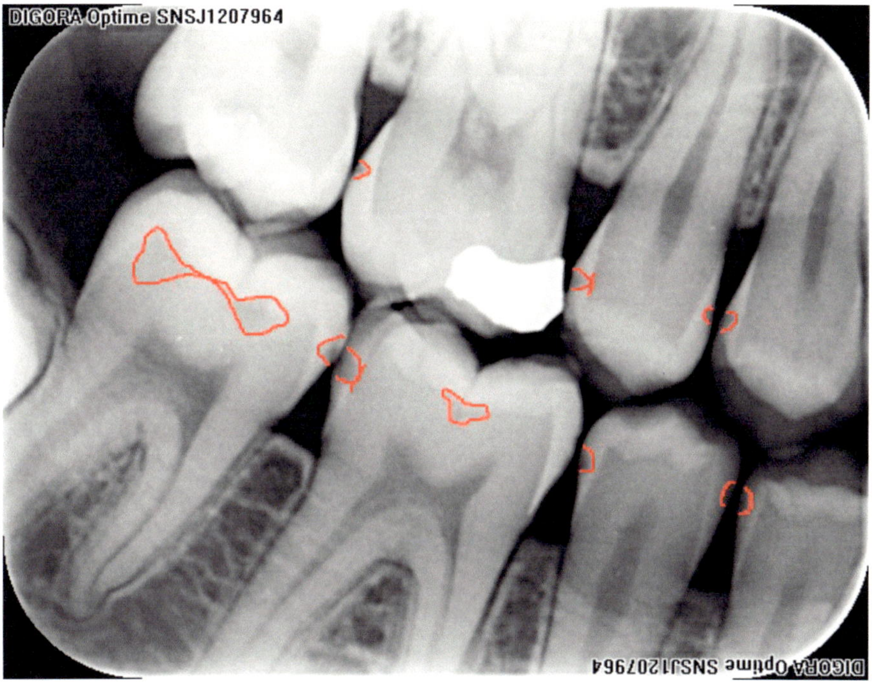


All the lesions seen in the previous x-ray are highlighted here.

*Let us test your knowledge to see what you have learnt*

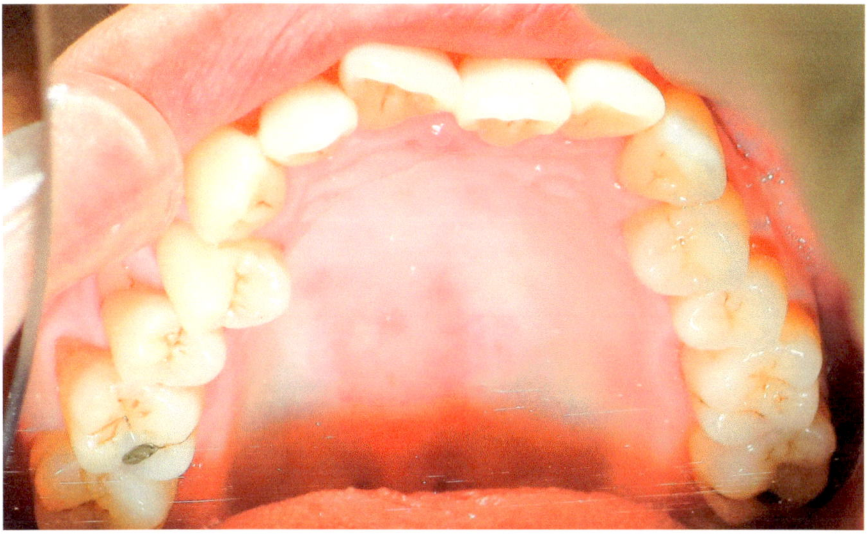

Test yourself - is there caries anywhere?

This page and the next six pages.

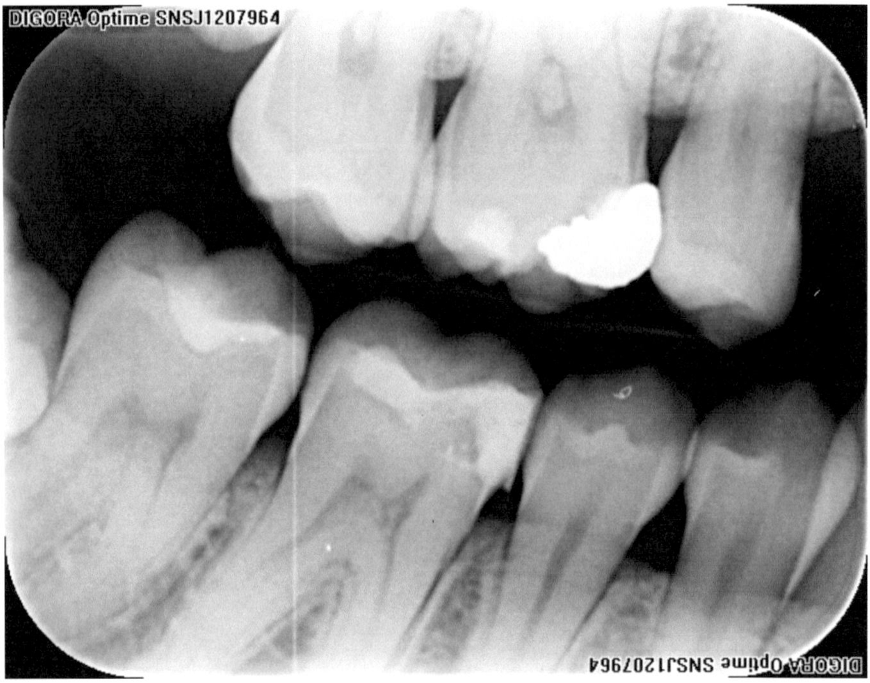


Spot the caries.

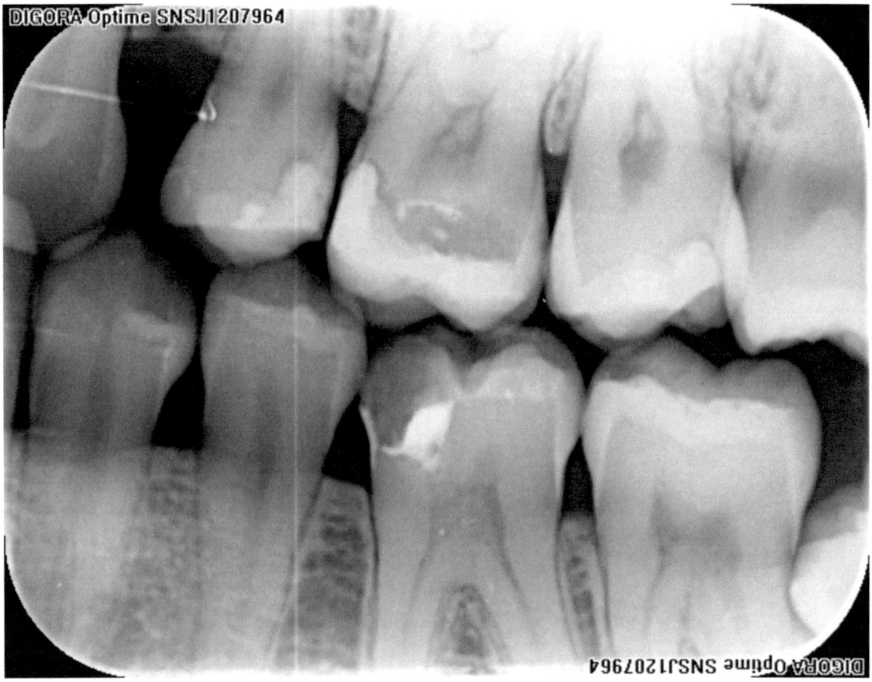


And again, spot the caries on these teeth.

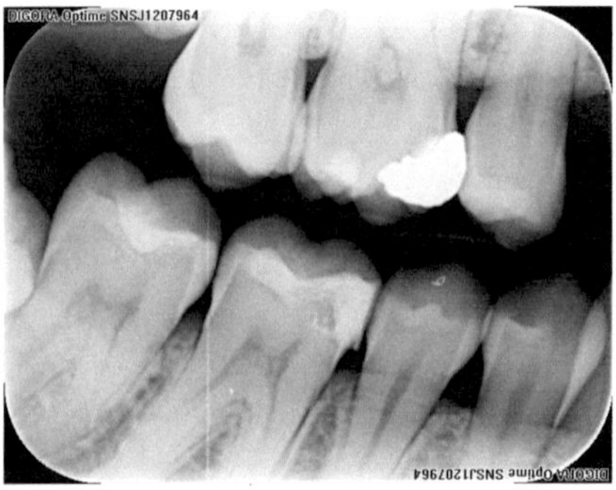


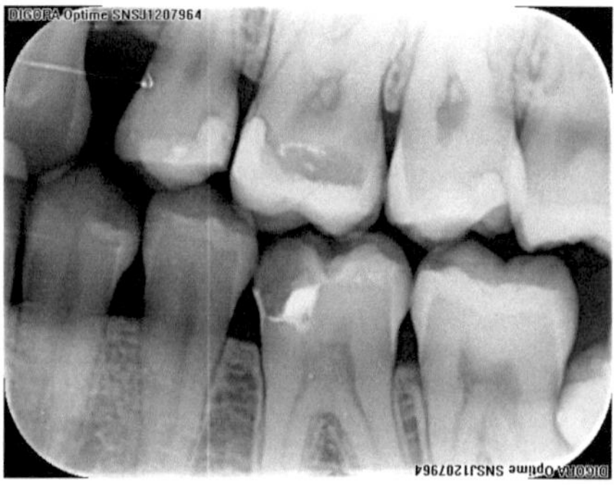


The patient is 21 years old with immaculate oral hygiene. My first thought when I saw this was "You poor thing, there is so much caries - have you not felt any pain or discomfort or sensitivity?" She has had no symptoms of any sort. I sent these bitewings to 3 colleagues, each with over 30 years' experience. We had no consensus, with views of "Yes, caries, lots of it", to "No caries". I decided I would investigate one of the teeth.

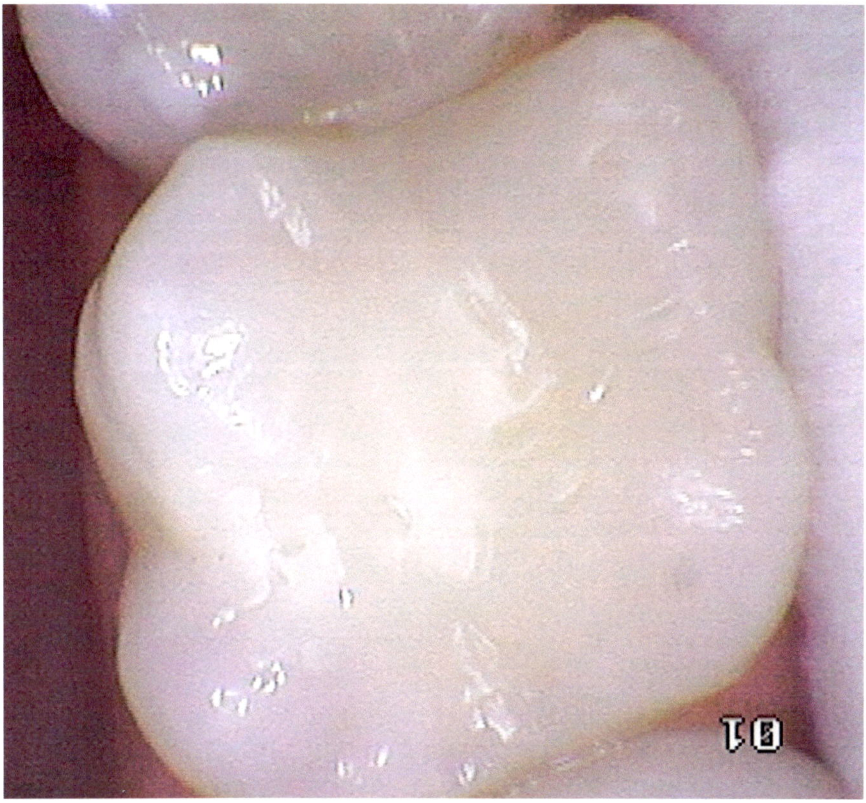

Tooth 26 before.

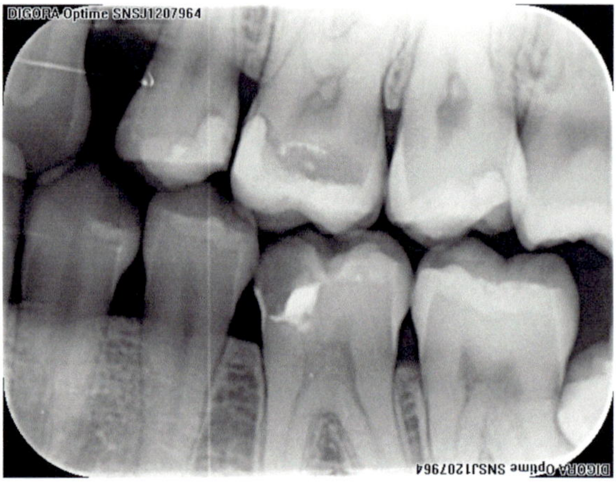


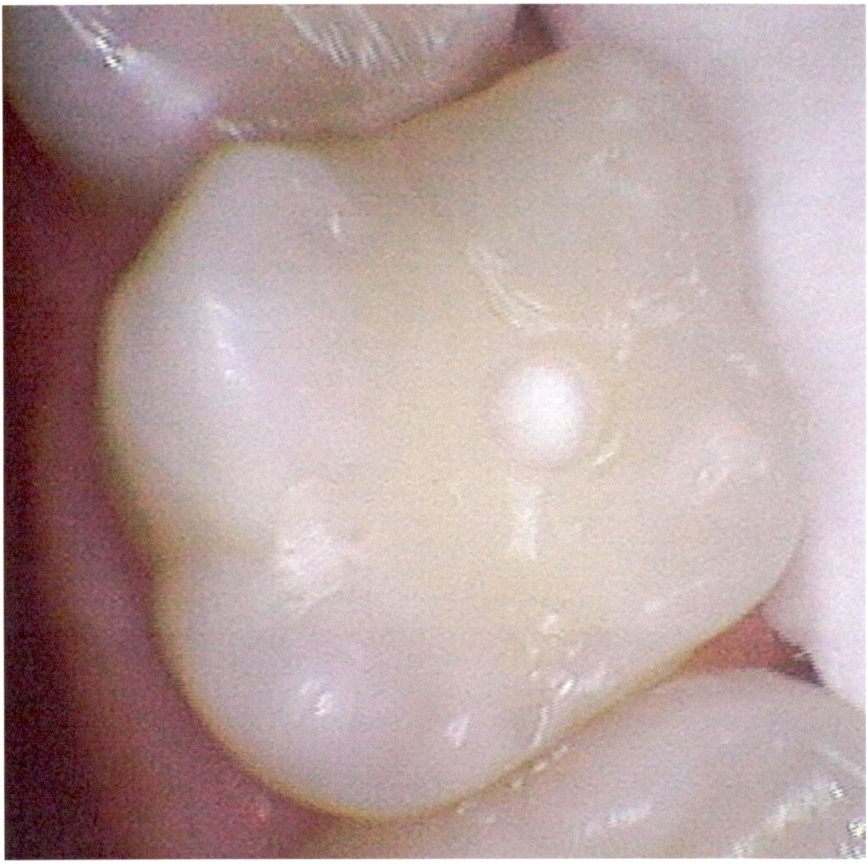

I drilled into 26, through the occlusal composite, and lo and behold! What do I see? A GIC base. Radiolucent on the x-ray.

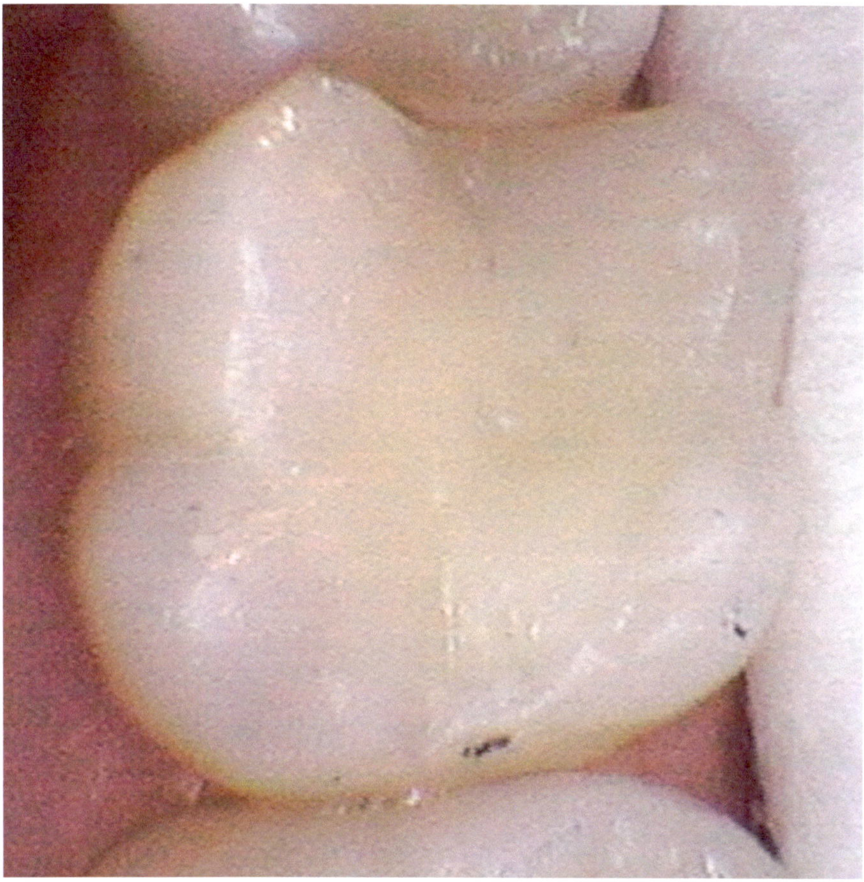

So I closed the investigative hole that I had made. Content. End of story.

Please do not use materials that are not radioopaque. Radiolucent materials could be mistaken for caries.

August 2015

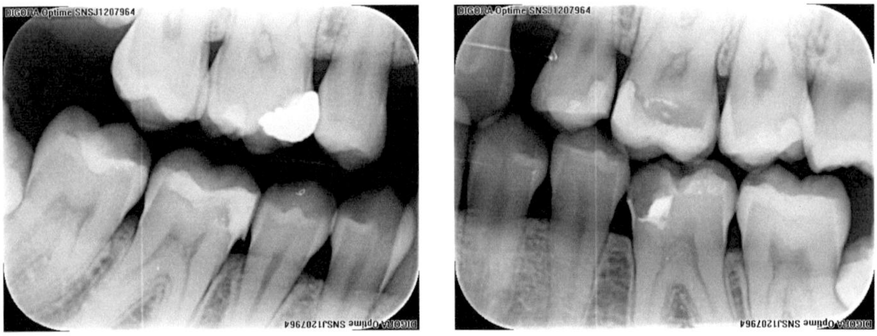


July 2017

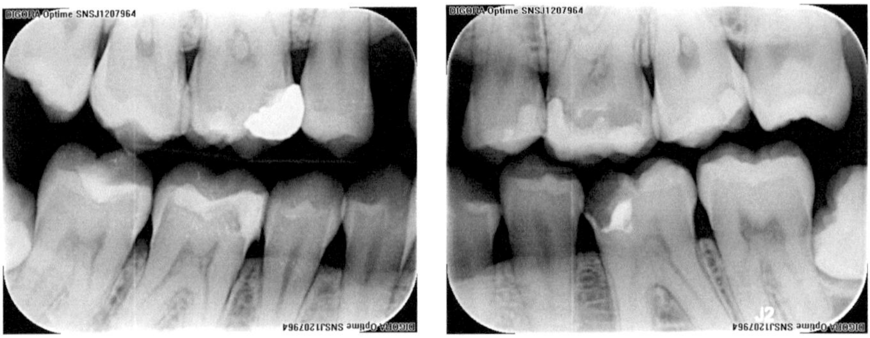


It turns out that there was a radiolucent base used beneath the fillings, giving the impression of caries beneath the fillings, when actually there was none.

# *Dental* CARIES

# AIDS IN DIAGNOSIS AND MANAGEMENT

# The First Few Minutes Spent With Your Patient

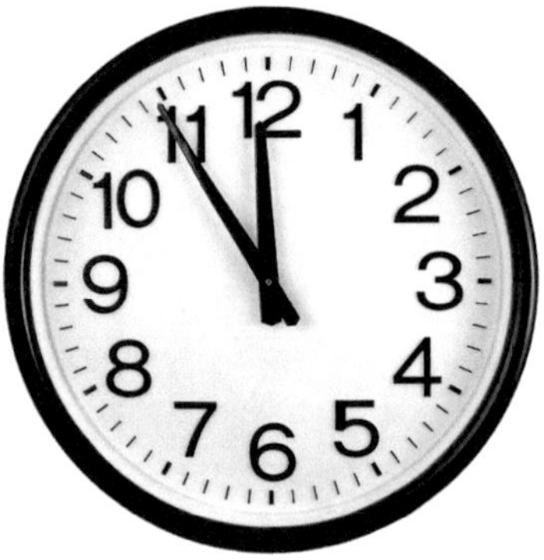


Make the patient comfortable, sitting up, in your dental chair.

Sit in front of the patient, face to face, without your mask on.

Try to be a little lower than your patient, rather than sitting higher than them.

Do not stand towering over the patient. Remember many patients are nervous to be in your surgery to begin with. Everything is strange to them. The clinical smells, the strange equipment, the intimidating instruments, the noises and the bright lighting seem more amplified to an anxious patient. Their senses are on edge and in overdrive.

Ask of the patient why they are here to see you. The few minutes you spend listening to the patient's symptoms and their response to your questions is time well spent. Very often this way you will have a good idea of what you can expect to see in the patient's mouth before you even lie them supine to have a look.

You will have obtained an idea of the patient's perception of dentists, whether they are regular attenders and care for their teeth together with regular visits to a dentist together with regular professional cleaning, or if they do not really want to be sitting opposite you and are only there because pain has finally forced them to seek help and who perhaps want knee-jerk responses to their problems.

# What to Listen Out For

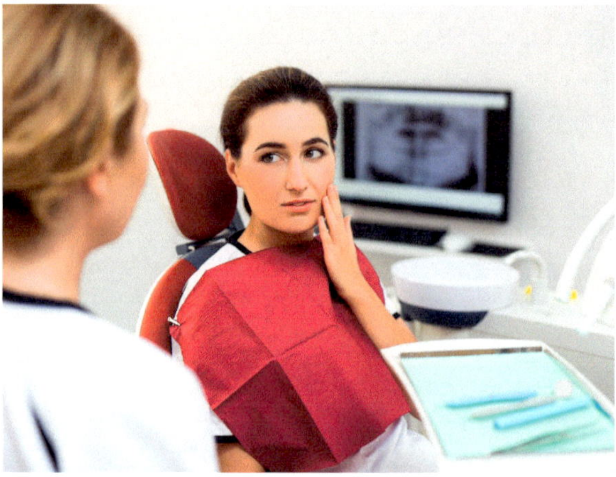

I have a tooth that is sensitive to cold and/or hot things

I have a tooth that reacts to sweet things

The sensitivity disappears straightaway/lingers for a while

The tooth aches constantly

The toothache is throbbing in nature

I cannot touch the tooth, it is sore to bite on

There is a swelling of the gum next to a tooth

The pain was intense but once the gum swelled up the pain became less

There has been a salty taste in my mouth from a tender/swollen gum

I am not sure whether my problem is from the upper or lower teeth

I know there is a hole in my tooth that has been there for a few years

My tooth broke a few days ago when I was eating

My tooth aches and I feel pain going up the side of my face

My tooth aches and I feel an ache along the lower jaw going past my ear

All the upper teeth on one/both sides are tender

I have this ache and the soreness goes away for a little while when I press my teeth together

I find if I hold lukewarm/tap water in the area it relieves the pain

There is a throbbing pain, it comes in waves, it wakes me up at night but I am not sure from which tooth

There is a throbbing pain and it is coming from THIS tooth

I bit on something hard, felt a crunch/crack and now it is sore when I bring my teeth together or move the broken tooth with my tongue.

# What to Look For

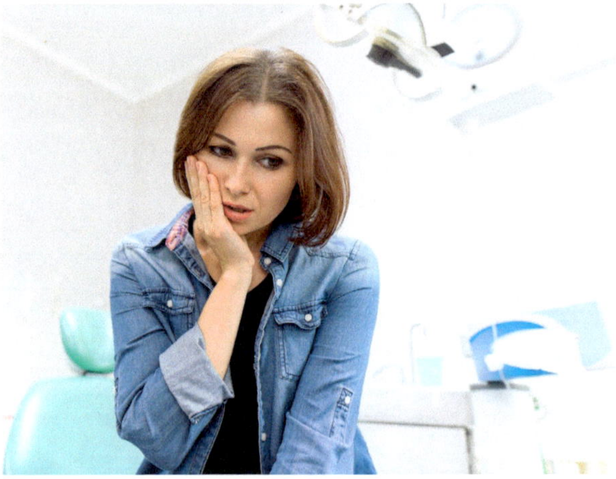

Is there swelling and tenderness of the submandibular or submental lymph nodes?

Does the patient have a bad head cold or blocked sinuses, or feel a heaviness in their head when they tilt their head forwards?

Ask the patient to point to where the problem is or even put their finger on the precise tooth.

Is there any facial swelling or intraoral swelling visible?

It is important to isolate the area with cotton wool rolls and to gently dry the area because most often it is those subtle changes in tooth colour that allow you to detect caries.

Most times the offending tooth is clear to spot when there is extensive caries.

Look for caries or a fracture. Has part of the tooth broken, commonly a thin cusp adjacent to a large (old) filling. Has that part broken away completely or is mobile and attached to the gingiva?

Compare the affected (sore) area with the (unaffected) contralateral area to compare differences in signs/sensation.

Press firmly against the alveolar bone close to the sulcus over a range of 3-4 teeth, opposite the root apices area, first on the unaffected side then equally firmly on the affected side. Is there a difference/tenderness? Go back to the affected side to localise it to a specific tooth. (If you suspect the problem is periodontal then press against the side of the teeth but closer to the gum line).

Push against the teeth buccal → palatal over a range of teeth, first on the unaffected side then on the affected side. Is there a difference/tenderness? Is there any "give" or mobility associated with the tenderness? Go back to the affected side to localise it to a specific tooth.

Percuss (tap) over a range of teeth, first on the unaffected side then on the affected side. Is there any soreness? Go back to the affected side to localise it to a specific tooth.

If there is barely or only a little tenderness to percussion and you suspect that there may be a crack in the tooth, percuss each cusp in turn and/or use a FracFinder.

Blow triplex air on where you think the problem is or over a range of teeth. If you get a false positive simply because of sensitive exposed root surface, then cover this area with a cotton roll and continue using triplex air to elicit symptoms. If no symptoms and you think the cause is as innocent as from exposed sensitive root surface, expose this area again, blow triplex air against it and ask the patient if that is EXACTLY the sensitivity they are experiencing. Rather than triplex air you could use a cold spray to do the same.

Ask the patient to sharply breathe in air to the sensitive area to see if the problem is from the exposed root surface/s.

To try to isolate a tooth that is reactive to hot stimuli, apply heat (e.g. warm gutta percha) on the teeth. Take care to protect the soft tissues from this heated gutta percha.

# What Do All the Symptoms and Signs Mean?

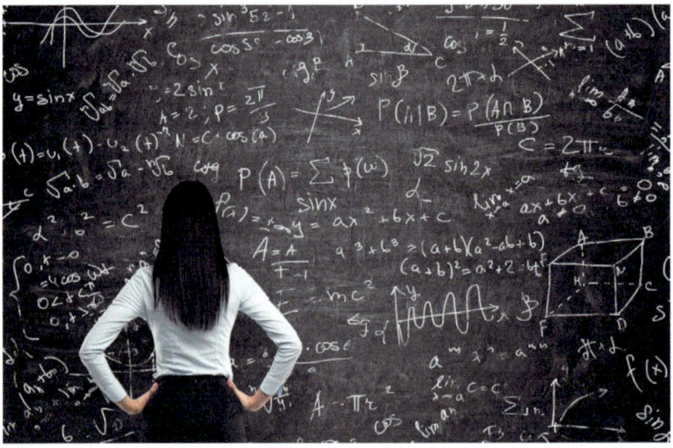

Sensitive to cold only, of recent onset.

More than likely needs just a filling.

Sensitive exposed root surface.

Either cover exposed area with a filling if the degree of wear or sensitivity is great, or, more conservatively, treat with desensitising agents such as Gluma, Bond or Duraphat, and advise easing off pressure on brushing, avoiding tangy and acidic fruits and juices and to use a desensitising toothpaste.

Sensitive to hot only or to both hot and cold.

Worries us more than sensitivity to cold alone. Usually indicates the problem is more extensive. Questioning patients will often reveal there have been symptoms for some time but are now bad enough to have driven the patients into your arms. There could well be pulpal involvement. Warn patient a filling alone may not work.

Sensitive to hot and cold (worse on hot) and ache at night.

Very high chance there is an irreversible pulpitis and that the pulp is on its way out. If you are going to try a filling only, warn the patient that this alone may not work, then be guided by where the caries takes you.

Sensitive to hot, relieved by holding tap water in mouth or pain relieved for a short period when presses teeth together.

Most likely irreversible pulpitis and discuss between endodontic treatment or extraction.

Throbbing pain, worse at night, stops patient from sleeping or wakes patient up at night.

A filling alone will not work. Discuss endodontic treatment, rebuild and crown (usually indicated) vs. extraction.

A thin part of the tooth has broken adjacent to an existing (and usually old) wide and large filling, no real discomfort unless the fractured portion is still there, mobile and attached to the gum.

Ideally crown but can "patch" so long as patient made aware this has variable prognosis and is a short term measure

Upper teeth on one side or both sides feel "different" or "tender" or 'dull". No raging toothache.

Ask if patient feels a heaviness in the head when bending forwards, has a bad head cold or suffers from sinusitis. If no other problems seen and a number of teeth feeling tender, consider the cause to be maxillary sinusitis.

**This is now perhaps 5-15 minutes into the patient's appointment time. Remember TIME IS OF THE ESSENCE. You have a pretty clear idea in your mind of what the treatment options are. You perhaps need to confirm this by taking intraoral radiographs (amongst other aids if deemed necessary) before discussing treatment options with the patient together with the costs involved.**

# Aids to Assist in Diagnosing

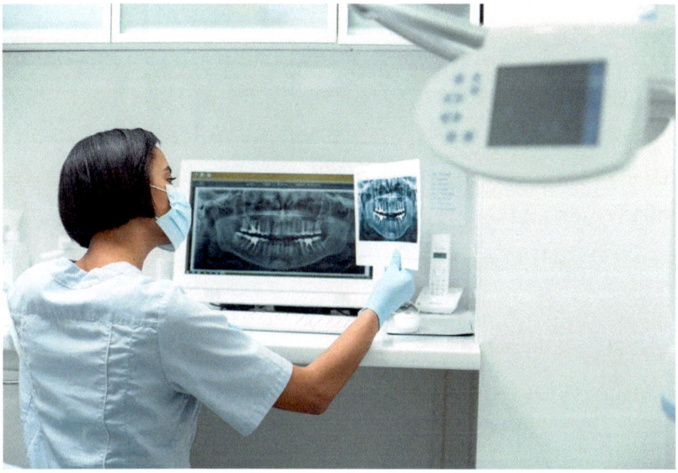

It is imperative that you conduct a careful and thorough examination of the affected region using your mouth mirror, probe/explorer together with the use of cotton wool rolls placed in the sulcus, allowing you to isolate the area and keep it dry, so as to detect those subtle changes in the colour of teeth that are indicative of disease.

If you feel the need is there, taking a Bitewing and, if needed, a Periapical radiograph will help.

For the Bitewing to be for any use it must be accurately taken:

Patient's occlusal plane parallel to the floor.
A 10° downward angle on the tube head.
The tube head positioned such that clear contacts are seen with no overlapping of the teeth where they touch each other. This is done by ensuring the tube head is 90° or perpendicular to the posterior teeth.

Digital radiographs using PSP plates are ideal as the image can be magnified and viewed in a multiple of formats and colour if required.

If the symptoms AND signs AND your investigations so far indicate the need, then periapical radiographs can help. Keep in mind that you are using ionising radiation and you need to keep patient (and you and your team) exposures to radiation to the minimum. The use of film holders used correctly assists greatly with accuracy, and hence with diagnostics.

A Panoramic / OPG radiograph may be called for
Testing the suspect area with Cold Spray if reactive to cold.
Testing the area with heated gutta percha if reactive to hot.
Testing the area with an electric pulp tester.
Transillumination to look for interstitial caries or cracks.
Using an intraoral camera.

# Treatment Provision

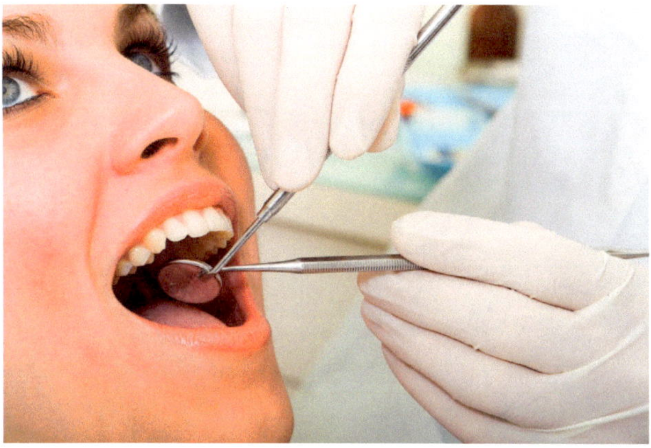

Are you clear on where the problem lies?

Does the tooth have caries and just a filling will work?

Is there secondary caries beneath a filling but you feel that just a filling will work?

Is the caries extensive and deep so that the tooth may require endodontic treatment or an extraction?

Is the tooth such that after you have filled it that the patient can expect a lingering sensitivity to cold for weeks after?

Will the tooth benefit by having a crown on it? Now? Later?

In dealing with caries or part of a tooth broken away in one part of a heavily filled tooth, will you undo all of the old filling or work "locally" only?

Does the age of the patient matter in your decision making?

# What to Do?

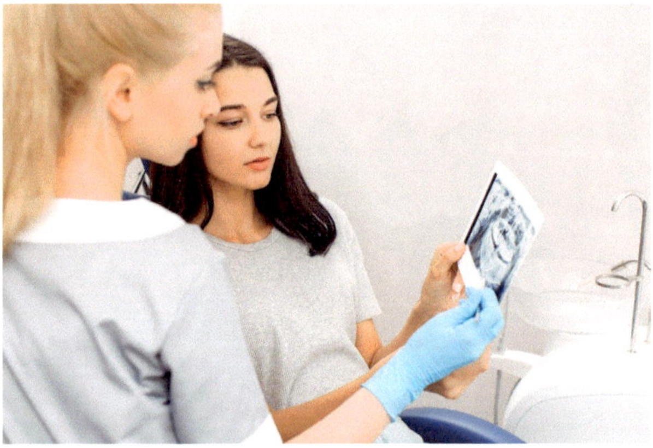

What does the patient want?

Remember the "customer is king".

Not everyone can afford endodontic treatment at approximately $800-1600 and a crown as well at $1500.

If the patient wants an extraction and it is not detrimental to their health, that's not the end of the world. Unlike eyes and ears and arms and legs, we have more than 2 teeth.

If you're talking to the patient about them spending $3000+ to save a tooth, in a mouth where there are many missing teeth, perhaps a denture is being worn, or 10-15 other teeth need attention, some maybe requiring extraction, whom are you doing a favour by asking the patient to spend this money on one tooth? What is the best option? Perhaps in this scenario your efforts should be directed to getting the patient comfortable and free of pain, and advise them that for their own good they should return for a comprehensive oral examination, discussion and holistic treatment planning.

You must inform the patient of all the treatment options and the associated costs. Then it is their call at the end of the day.

# Other Considerations

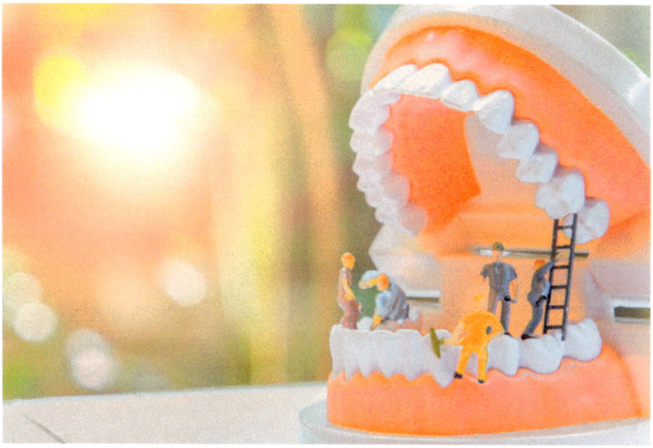

If you advocate replacing a large MODP amalgam filling on 16 with a resin restoration because the thin dp cusp has broken away and there are no symptoms apart from a rough edge worrying the tongue and there is no caries, on a 70 year old patient where the filling is about 55 years old, will your filling be better or equal to what has served him/her so well for so long? Will you establish good tight contacts to replicate what this amalgam filling had successfully done, so that you do not create entirely new issues/problems of food packing? Are you better off just rounding off sharp edges if there is no risk of caries? Should you go straight to a crown?

If you see stained fissures in a 50-60 year old who has had no new caries or problems for years, has decent oral hygiene and periodontal health, why do anything?

Conversely, if you see plaque filled fissures in just erupted second molars of a 12 year old in whom all the first molars have already had to be filled and whose mouth rarely sees a toothbrush, it may be prudent to seal those fissures as quickly as you can.

You know that amalgam fillings expand on setting. Often at the filling/tooth junction on the occlusal surface enamel prisms break away leading to "ditching". This alone does not mean that you need to replace the filling.

You know that composite resin fillings contract on setting, so when you see discolouration at the filling/tooth junction, in the absence of caries, you need not do anything. This discolouration may easily polish away if the filling is not flush with the tooth.

If in your mouth we took out alternate teeth, on the mesial and distal surfaces of the teeth that remain there will be staining at the contact areas. And that is all it is. Staining, plain and simple. Nothing for you to go hacking into. If the enamel surfaces have caved in or crumbled in these areas, this is where you make a decision as to where you drill and clean and fill, or do nothing. If the area has been like that for 20 years on an 80 year old (with a tiny cavity, tooth hard and dark) compared to a small mesial area of breakdown, light in colour at the base, in a 12 year old where the "E" has just been shed, your approach to managing each of these should be different.

# Checklist

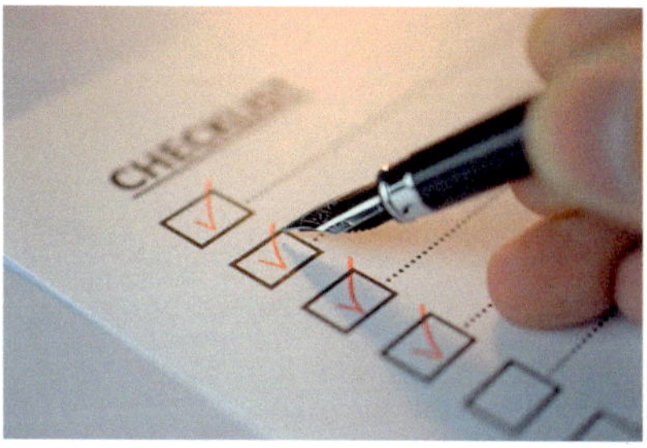


Have you determined the cause of the sensitivity or pain?

Do you know exactly where the cause of pain/symptoms lies?

Have you explained all the treatment options and possible sequelae to the patient?

Have you explained the treatment costs to the patient?

Is the treatment to be provided within your expertise?

Remember, First Do No Harm.

# What to Warn the Patient About

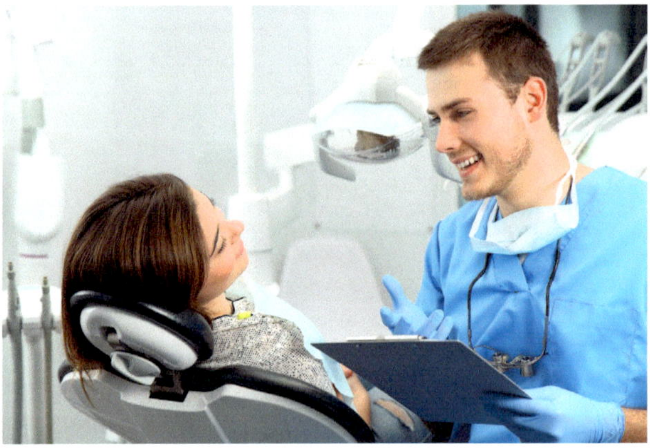

Depending on the circumstances, symptoms, what you had to do and how extensive the problem was:

If the cavity was really deep and close to the pulp.

If there was a carious exposure of the pulp and you placed a pulp cap.

If there is a crack line involving a corner of the tooth or running along the entire floor of the cavity.

Then warn the patient that the tooth may have sensitivity to cold things for some time after. If you anticipate that the sensitivity will settle, advise them. Likewise, if you think it may not, similarly advise them.

Caution the patient that the tooth may require endodontic treatment.

Advise the patient that part of the remaining tooth structure is thin and may break over time.

Advise the patient that the tooth ideally requires a crown to go on as a glove or sleeve over it to protect it from breakdown.

If need be tell the patient that you have done the best that you could do and that the outlook for the tooth is not good.

Do tell the patient that nothing lasts forever, and that even with the most optimal oral hygiene that a new large resin restoration may not stand up to their chewing forces.

**Excerpt from ADA News Bulletin May 2017 No 464 Clinical Performance of resin-based composite in posterior teeth**

Microfilled composites do not perform as well as hybrid composites.

AFR (annual failure rate) of 3.1% mainly due to bulk fractures and secondary caries.

Of composite failures 74% were due to secondary caries, 8% due to total loss and 5.3% due to fracture.

Failure rates increase as the number of restored surfaces increases. The more surfaces restored the greater the chance of reduced longevity.

Higher failure rate in patients over 65 years of age.

Post operative sensitivity is not much of an issue any more due to improvements in adhesive bonding systems.

The overall long term success of the restorations has improved even though more complex restorations are being placed.

Overall must take care to control the oral environment during restoration placement and care taken to follow the manufacturer's instructions correctly.

Martin Tyas
Dental Instruments, Materials and Equipment Committee
Australian Dental Association.
ADA News Bulletin May 2017 No 464

# What Never to Tell Patients

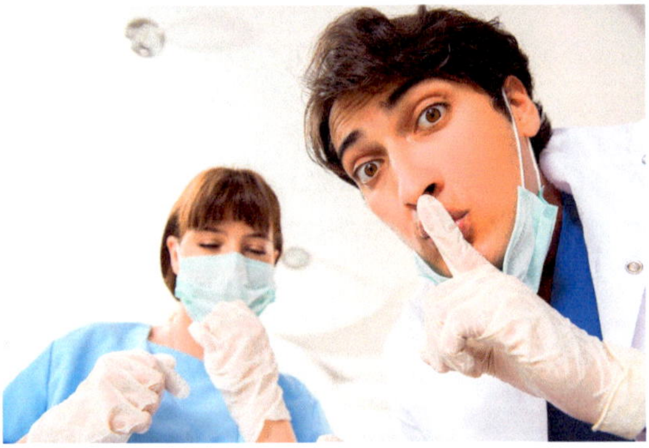

That your work will last forever.

That everything will be fine when you know there is a chance it may not be.

Do not openly criticize work done in their mouth that you see because you do not know the circumstances under which it was done. The patient might be telling you one thing but remember that there are always two sides to a story.

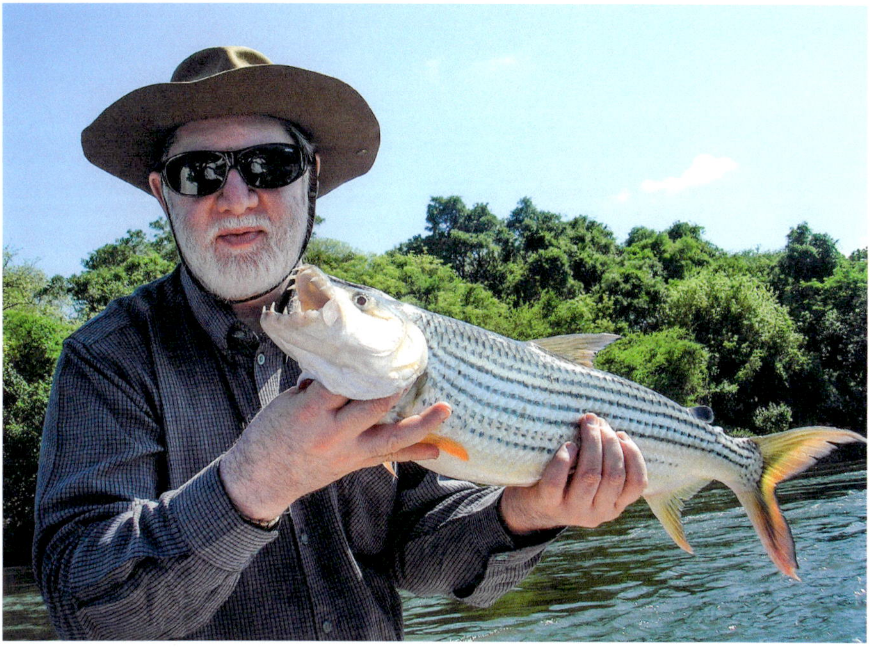

The author's passion outside of dentistry. The tiger fish is native to only a few river systems in southern Africa

Tiger Fish, Zambesi River, Chirundu, Zimbabwe

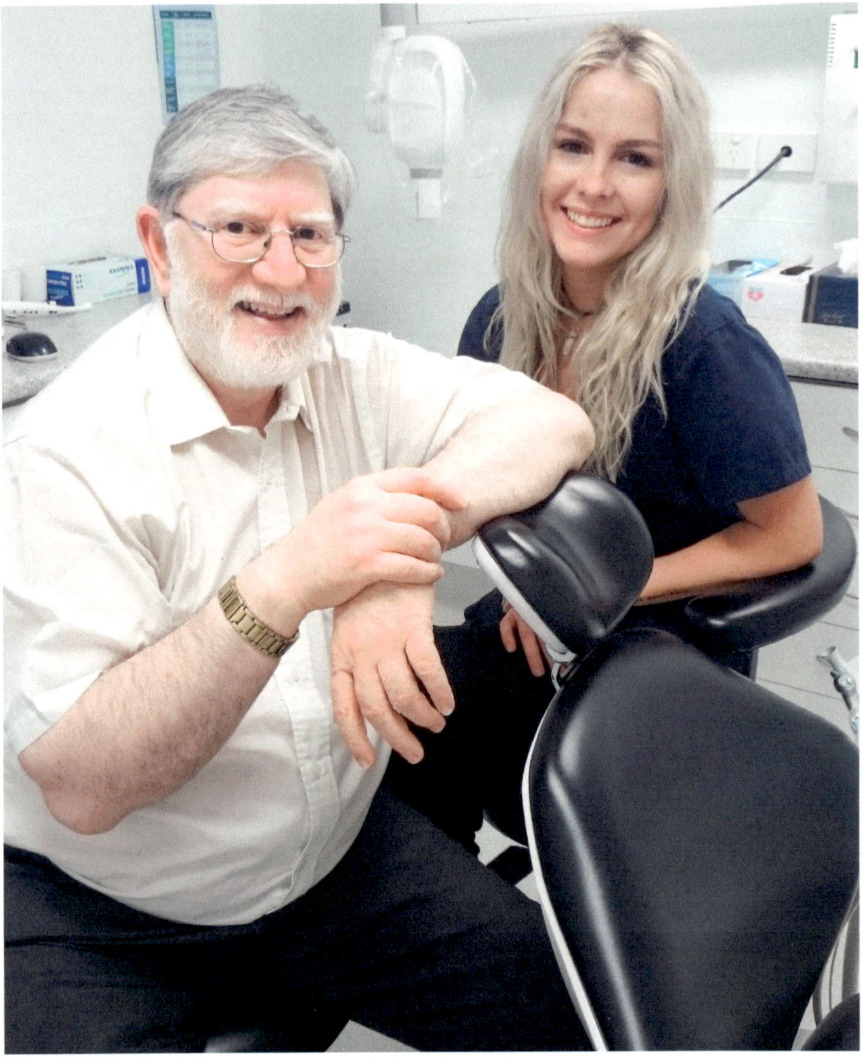

*An Atlas of Dental Caries*

A Pictorial For Dental Students and Dentists

is also available on Amazon Kindle as an eBook

For educational resources for dental students
and junior dentists, visit:

www.mydentaleducation.com

Look out for other books in this series.

Made in the USA
Monee, IL
12 July 2026

57049286R00128